Statistics and Informatics in Molecular Cancer Research

Statistics and Informatics in Molecular Cancer Research

Edited by

Carsten Wiuf
Bioinformatics Research Center, Aarhus University

Claus L. Andersen
Department of Molecular Medicine, Aarhus University Hospital

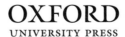

OXFORD
UNIVERSITY PRESS

Great Clarendon Street, Oxford OX2 6DP

Oxford University Press is a department of the University of Oxford.
It furthers the University's objective of excellence in research, scholarship,
and education by publishing worldwide in

Oxford New York

Auckland Cape Town Dar es Salaam Hong Kong Karachi
Kuala Lumpur Madrid Melbourne Mexico City Nairobi
New Delhi Shanghai Taipei Toronto

With offices in

Argentina Austria Brazil Chile Czech Republic France Greece
Guatemala Hungary Italy Japan Poland Portugal Singapore
South Korea Switzerland Thailand Turkey Ukraine Vietnam

Oxford is a registered trade mark of Oxford University Press
in the UK and in certain other countries

Published in the United States
by Oxford University Press Inc., New York

© Oxford University Press 2009

The moral rights of the authors have been asserted
Database right Oxford University Press (maker)

First Published 2009

All rights reserved. No part of this publication may be reproduced,
stored in a retrieval system, or transmitted, in any form or by any means,
without the prior permission in writing of Oxford University Press,
or as expressly permitted by law, or under terms agreed with the appropriate
reprographics rights organization. Enquiries concerning reproduction
outside the scope of the above should be sent to the Rights Department,
Oxford University Press, at the address above

You must not circulate this book in any other binding or cover
and you must impose the same condition on any acquirer

British Library Cataloguing in Publication Data
Data available

Library of Congress Cataloging in Publication Data
Data available

Typeset by Newgen Imaging Systems (P) Ltd., Chennai, India
Printed in Great Britain
on acid-free paper by
Clays Ltd, St Ives Plc

ISBN 978–0–19–953287–2

1 3 5 7 9 10 8 6 4 2

CONTENTS

Preface   x
References   xii

1   Association studies   1
    Emily Webb and Richard Houlston

    1.1   Introduction   1
    1.2   Sequence variation and patterns of linkage disequilibrium in the genome   2
    1.3   Direct and indirect association studies   4
    1.4   Preliminary analysis and quality control   5
        1.4.1   Assessment of call rates   5
        1.4.2   Duplicate samples   6
        1.4.3   Relatedness between study subjects   6
        1.4.4   Hardy–Weinberg equilibrium   6
        1.4.5   Quantile–quantile plots   7
    1.5   Techniques for detecting association   7
        1.5.1   Single locus tests   7
        1.5.2   Incorporating covariates   9
        1.5.3   Multi-locus tests   10
        1.5.4   Interactive and additive effects   11
        1.5.5   Pathway analysis   12
        1.5.6   Subgroup analysis   12
        1.5.7   Imputation of genotypes   13
        1.5.8   Confounding and stratification   13
    1.6   Statistical power and multiple testing   14
        1.6.1   Design strategies for increasing power   16
        1.6.2   The staged design   17
    1.7   Replication, quantification, and identification of causal variants   17
    1.8   Discussion   18
    1.9   URLs   19
    References   20

2   Methods for DNA copy number derivations   25
    Cameron Brennan

    2.1   Copy number aberration in cancer   25
    2.2   Obtaining and analysing copy number data: platforms and initial processing   25
        2.2.1   Array-CGH   26

		2.2.2	Oligonucleotide arrays	26
		2.2.3	Representational methods	28
		2.2.4	Digital karyotyping and sequencing-based approaches	28
	2.3	Choosing a platform: array resolution and practical considerations		29
	2.4	Segmentation		31
		2.4.1	Artifacts	33
	2.5	Aberration types		34
		2.5.1	Regional and focal aberrations	34
		2.5.2	Copy number variation	36
		2.5.3	Regional/broad CNA	37
		2.5.4	Focal CNA	37
	2.6	Assigning significance to CNA		39
	2.7	Breakpoints/translocations		44
	2.8	Clustering approaches		46
	2.9	Conclusion		48
	References			48
3	Methods for derivation of LOH and allelic copy numbers using SNP arrays			52
	Carsten Wiuf, Philippe Lamy and Claus L. Andersen			
	3.1	Introduction		52
		3.1.1	Overview	53
		3.1.2	Retinoblastoma	53
		3.1.3	Identification of TSGs	54
		3.1.4	Mechanisms causing AI (in particular LOH)	54
		3.1.5	Genomic alterations and their relation to clinical end-points	55
	3.2	Experimental determination of LOH		56
	3.3	SNP genotyping arrays		57
		3.3.1	Normalization	57
		3.3.2	Genotyping	58
	3.4	Simple computational tools to infer LOH		60
		3.4.1	Classification of genotypes	60
		3.4.2	Regions with same boundary (RSB)	60
		3.4.3	Nearest Neighbour (NN)	61
	3.5	Advanced statistical tools for LOH inference		61
		3.5.1	Hidden Markov models	61
		3.5.2	Example	63
		3.5.3	Two main problems	65
		3.5.4	An interpretation of the hidden Markov model	65
		3.5.5	Limitations to the HMM approach	65
	3.6	Estimation of allele specific copy numbers		67
		3.6.1	An allele specific HMM	68
		3.6.2	Normalization	68

	3.6.3	The states	70
	3.6.4	Example	70
3.7	Conclusion		74
References			74

4 Bioinformatics of gene expression and copy number data integration   78
   Outi Monni and Sampsa Hautaniemi

4.1	Introduction		78
4.2	Methods		79
	4.2.1	Methods to study copy number levels	79
	4.2.2	Methods to study gene expression	80
	4.2.3	Microarrays in detection of copy number and gene expression levels	81
4.3	Microarray experiment		81
4.4	Analysis and integration of gene expression and copy number data		87
	4.4.1	Preprocessing	87
	4.4.2	Identifying amplified and deleted regions from array-CGH data	89
	4.4.3	Statistical approach to integrate gene expression and array-CGH data	90
	4.4.4	Data reduction model approach to integrate gene expression and array-CGH data	94
	4.4.5	Interpolation	96
	4.4.6	Gene annotation	97
4.5	Conclusions		97
References			98

5 Analysis of DNA methylation in cancer   102
   Fabian Model, Jörn Lewin, Catherine Lofton-Day and
   Gunter Weiss

5.1	Introduction		102
	5.1.1	DNA methylation biology	102
	5.1.2	DNA methylation in cancer	103
	5.1.3	Overview	105
5.2	Measuring DNA methylation		105
	5.2.1	Measurement technologies	105
	5.2.2	Quantification of DNA methylation	108
5.3	Data preprocessing		109
	5.3.1	Direct bisulphite sequencing	110
	5.3.2	DNA microarrays	114
5.4	Data analysis		118
	5.4.1	Tissue classification using DNA microarrays	118
	5.4.2	Plasma based cancer detection	123
	5.4.3	Cancer recurrence prediction	126

	5.5	Conclusions	128
	References		128
6	Pathway analysis: Pathway signatures and classification		132
	Ming Yi and Robert M. Stephens		
	6.1	Overview of pathway analysis	132
		6.1.1 Pathway and network visualization methods	132
		6.1.2 Gene-set based methods	136
	6.2	From gene signatures/classifiers to pathway signatures/classifiers	138
		6.2.1 Gene signature and classifiers	138
		6.2.2 Pathway signatures/classifiers as an alternative?	140
		6.2.3 Current advances in pathway-level signatures and pathway classification	142
	6.3	Potentials of pathway-based analysis for integrative discovery	147
	6.4	Conclusions	151
	References		152
7	Two methods for comparing genomic data across independent studies in cancer research: Meta-analysis and oncomine concepts map		160
	Wendy Lockwood Banka, Matthew J. Anstett and Daniel R. Rhodes		
	7.1	Introduction	160
	7.2	Single-study gene expression analyses in oncomine	161
		7.2.1 Differential expression analysis	161
		7.2.2 Co-expression analysis	163
	7.3	Meta-analysis	164
	7.4	Application	164
	7.5	Oncomine concepts map	167
		7.5.1 Assembling gene signatures	167
		7.5.2 Association analysis	168
	7.6	Application	169
		7.6.1 Direct comparison of oncomine concepts results to meta-analysis results	169
	7.7	Conclusion	174
	References		174
8	Bioinformatic approaches to the analysis of alternative splicing variants in cancer biology		177
	Lue Ping Zhao, Jessica Andriesen and Wenhong Fan		
	8.1	Introduction to alternative splicing	177
		8.1.1 Traditional methods for splicing analysis	177
		8.1.2 Current estimates of alternative splicing in humans	179
		8.1.3 Alternative splicing and cancer	179

8.2		onucleotide arrays for detecting alternative cing variants	179
	8.2.1	cDNA arrays	180
	8.2.2	GeneChip arrays	180
	8.2.3	GeneChip exon arrays	181
	8.2.4	Tiling arrays	181
8.3	Bioin	formatic approaches	182
	8.3.1	Two group design	182
	8.3.2	Functional alternative splicing variants utilizing exon arrays	183
	8.3.3	A general framework	184
	8.3.4	Relative versus absolute abundance	186
	8.3.5	Detection limits	187
8.4	An ex	xample	187
8.5	Futur	re directions	189
References		190

Index   193

PREFACE

Molecular understanding of cancer and cancer progression is at the forefront of many research programmes today. High-throughput array technologies and other modern molecular techniques produce a wealth of molecular data about the structure, organization, and function of cells, tissues and organisms. Correctly analysed and interpreted these data hold the promise of bringing new markers for prognostic and diagnostic use, for new treatment schemes, and of gaining new biological insight into the evolution of cancer and its molecular, pathological and clinical consequences. For these purposes, however, mathematical, statistical and bioinformatics tools (in short: informatics tools) are urgently needed to extract, handle and process the information in the data, and to assist in planning of future experiments.

At one level cancer is a simple disease – the diagnose is typically a clear-cut question of yes or no – at the molecular and pathological level, though, cancer is a highly heterogeneous disease and even tissue-specific cancers show a high level of heterogeneity phenotypically as well as molecularly. Cancer arises from multiple genetic or epigenetic lesions that are accompanied by changes in numerous processes, including DNA repair, cellular proliferation, cell-cycle control and apoptosis. Dysregulation of the complex interplay between genes taking part in these processes can ultimately lead to tumorgenesis. Molecularly, cancer diseases are different from most other diseases in that they involve dramatic changes at the DNA, RNA and higher information levels that seldom (if ever) are seen to the same extent in other diseases.

High-throughput technologies, in particular microarray technologies, have dramatically transformed molecular biology and medicine. Within a single experiment it is possible to measure millions of molecular variables simultaneously and relate the variables to molecular and clinical parameters (such as molecular phenotypes and clinical outcomes). This has changed molecular medicine from focusing on a single or few features (e.g. genes or markers) to focusing on sets of features, signatures and pathways derived by a combination of data-mining, statistics and bioinformatics. In this way, we see the cell or organism as a system where individual components alone may contribute little to the functioning and activities of the system, but in conjunction with other components they may be key or essential players.

This transformation of molecular medicine requires new statistics and informatics tools to search or mine data, and to identify features or groups of features that statistically appear extraordinary in some sense. For example, several studies have identified gene signatures that reliably differentiate between subgroups or stages of cancers (Golub *et al.*, 1999; van't Veer *et al.*, 2002; Dyrskjøt *et al.*,

2005). Such signatures or classifiers have an obvious diagnostic and prognostic potential, but also provide new biological insight into cancer progression and aethiology (Clarke *et al.*, 2008; Lakhani and Ashworth, 2001).

From the mid-1990s where the first DNA microarray technologies became commercially available and until today, the amount and quality of the data collected in an array experiment have improved immensely. The first Affymetrix GeneChip® SNP array, released in 1995, contained approximately 1500 unique single nucleotide polymorphisms (SNPs) in the human genome – thirteen years later Affymetrix, Illumina and other SNP arrays contain well over a million SNPs. Likewise the first RNA expression microarrays targeted roughly 10,000 genes in the human genome – today they target more than 50,000 known and predicted genes/transcripts. Part of the story is the completion of the Human Genome Project in 2000 that made the first realiable human genome sequence available. With that at hand the genome could be covered much more extensively with probes measuring DNA and RNA abundance than previously had been possible. Subsequent refinements of the genome build have resulted in improved genomic coordinates of the probes and improved knowledge of the genomic context they are in. Alongside these technological advances this has resulted in high-performance array technologies.

However, part of the success of high-throughput technologies is also advances in informatics. Since the release of the first array technologies statisticians and bioinformaticians all over the world have been interested in developing methods for analysing and extracting information from array data. Naturally, to cope with a high level of molecular complexity non-standard informatics tools are required. This has resulted in new theoretical and practical development in informatics and in increased collaboration between old disciplines. Some tools are developed specifically for cancer research, while others are applicable in many different situations.

It is the aim of this book to make the bioinformatics tools used for cancer research available to a wide range of researchers, in a single coherent volume – covering the theory behind the tools and their application to real data. Traditionally, one distinguishes between high and low level analysis, where low level analysis refers to normalization of the data before a (high-level) biologically relevant analysis can be done. Normalization comprises removing background and technology related/specific noise that otherwise would make comparison of data across experiments difficult. The focus of the book is high-level analysis. Naturally, it takes many forms that depend on the technology platform applied and the biology one wants to uncover. The book presents examples of analysis of many types of data, from DNA, to RNA and methylation data, their combination and how additional data from other data sets or databases can facilitate more detailed and powerful analysis.

Claus L. Andersen
Aarhus University Hospital

Carsten Wiuf
Aarhus University

References

Clarke, R., Ressom, H.W., Wang, A., Xuan, J., Liu, M.C., Gehan, E.A., and Wang, Y. (2008). The properties of high-dimensional data spaces: implications for exploring gene and protein expression data. *Nature Reviews Cancer*, **8**, 37–49.

Dyrskjøt, L., Zieger, K., Kruhffer, M., Thykjaer, T., Jensen, J. L., Primdahl, H., Aziz, N., Marcussen, N., Møller, K., and Orntoft, T.F. (2005). A molecular signature in superficial bladder carcinoma predicts clinical outcome. *Clin. Cancer Res.*, **11**, 4029–4036.

Golub, T.R., Slonim, D.K., Tamayo, P., Huard, C., Gaasenbeek, M., Mesirov, J.P., Coller, H., Loh, M.L., Downing, J.R., Caligiuri, M.A., Bloomfield, C.D., and Lander, E.S. (1999). Molecular classification of cancer: class discovery and class prediction by gene expression monitoring. *Science*, **286**, :531–537.

Lakhani, S.R. and Ashworth, A. (2001). Microarray and histopathological analysis of tumours: the future and the past? *Nature Reviews Cancer*, **1**, 151–157.

van't Veer, L.J., Dai, H., van de Vijver, M.J., He, Y.D., Hart, A.A., Mao, M., Peterse, H.L., van der Kooy, K., Marton, M.J., Witteveen, A.T., Schreiber, G.J., Kerkhoven, R.M., Roberts, C., Linsley, P.S., Bernards, R., and Friend, S.H. (2002). Gene expression profiling predicts clinical outcome of breast cancer. *Nature*, **415**, 530–536.

1
ASSOCIATION STUDIES

Emily Webb and Richard Houlston

1.1 Introduction

Until recently, research on inherited cancer susceptibility has principally focused on the identification of mutations segregating with disease in large families. Genetic linkage analysis coupled with positional cloning has proved to be a highly efficient strategy for the discovery of cancer genes and led to the identification of highly penetrant genes for a number of common cancers, including breast and ovarian cancers (*BRCA1* and *BRCA2* on chromosomes 17 and 13; Hall *et al.* 1990; Wooster *et al.* 1994), colon cancer with adenomatous polyposis coli (*APC* on chromosome 5; Bodmer *et al.* 1987), hereditary non-polyposis colorectal cancer (the mismatch repair genes *MSH2* and *MLH1* on chromosomes 2 and 3; Lindblom *et al.* 1993; Peltomaki *et al.* 1993), and melanoma (*CDNK2A* on chromosome 9; Cannon-Albright *et al.* 1992).

Twin studies indicate that for most of the common cancers, much of the familial aggregation of disease results from inherited susceptibility (Lichtenstein *et al.*, 2000), for example, 27% of breast, 35% of colorectal and 42% of prostate cancers. Highly penetrant mutations in known genes, however, cannot account for most of the excess familial risk of these tumours, for example mutations in known predisposition genes *BRCA1* and *BRCA2*, account for only ∼20% of the two-fold excess risk in breast cancer patients' relatives (Anglian Breast Cancer Study Group, 2000). Similarly, only ∼3% of colorectal cancer can be ascribed to germline mutations in *APC*, *MLH1* or *MSH2* and for prostate cancer, mutations in *BRCA2* account for only ∼2% of early-onset disease. The remaining familial risk could be due to high-penetrance mutations in as yet unidentified genes, but multiple-case cancer families segregating none of the known mutations have failed to reveal significant linkage to novel loci in recent studies, and a polygenic mechanism now appears more plausible (Peto 2002; Pharoah *et al.* 2002; Antoniou and Easton 2003). Under the polygenic model or 'common-disease common-variant' hypothesis, a large number of common alleles each conferring a small genotypic risk (typically 1.1–1.5) combine additively or multiplicatively to confer a range of susceptibilities in the population. Individuals carrying few such alleles would be at reduced risk while those with many might suffer a lifetime risk as high as 50% (Fig. 1.1). If low-penetrance alleles cause a substantial proportion of this inherited susceptibility to cancer, their identification is of great practical importance.

Alleles that increase cancer incidence by two-fold or less will rarely cause multiple-case families and are therefore difficult or impossible to identify through

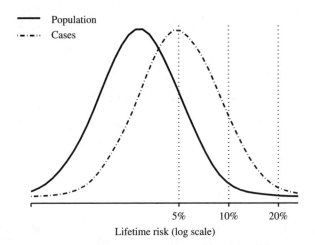

FIG. 1.1: The polygenic model of cancer risk. Distribution of lifetime cancer risk in the general population (solid line) and in individuals who will develop cancer (dashed line).

linkage (Risch and Merikangas, 1996). For example, to detect a gene with frequency 0.1 conferring a two-fold increase in risk by linkage would require about 10,000 affected sibling pairs. In contrast, it should be detectable through association, where the frequencies of genetic variants are compared in cases and controls, with only 500 unselected cases and 500 controls. The search for low-penetrance alleles has therefore centred increasingly on association studies.

Recent data from genome-wide association studies (GWAS) of prostate, breast and colorectal cancer (Amundadottir *et al.* 2006; Easton *et al.* 2007; Tomlinson *et al.* 2007) have vindicated the 'common-disease common-variant' hypothesis and indicate that such studies provide a highly efficient strategy for identifying novel disease loci and gaining further understanding of the allelic architecture of inherited susceptibility to cancer.

In this chapter we first introduce the biological principles underlying association studies. We then discuss preliminary statistical analysis and quality control measures before describing the statistical techniques used to search for disease associations. Finally, we review power and study design considerations and give a brief overview of the steps required to move from association study discovery to elucidation of causal variant. The theory and techniques described throughout the chapter are illustrated with specific reference to the field of cancer; however they may equally be applied to association studies for any complex disease.

1.2 Sequence variation and patterns of linkage disequilibrium in the genome

Single nucleotide polymorphisms (SNPs) are by far the most common form of polymorphic variation in the human genome, with an estimated 10 million SNPs, collectively accounting for over 90% of sequence variation (Botstein and Risch, 2003). A SNP is a DNA sequence variation that occurs when a single nucleotide in the genome varies between two individuals or between paired chromosomes in the same individual. Each SNP has two alleles, the original sequence (wild type allele) and the mutated copy. A person's genotype defined by a specific SNP can therefore be WW, WM, or MM; where W and M correspond to wild type and mutated sequences, respectively.

Single nucleotide polymorphisms can be categorized on the basis of their location in the genome. While the vast majority of SNPs map to untranslated regions of the genome, a small proportion localize to coding regions. A minority of these coding SNPs (cSNPs) alter the encoded amino acid sequence (non-synonymous SNPs; nsSNPs). Such nsSNPs are proportionally less prevalent than synonymous SNPs, which do not alter protein sequence, possibly as a consequence of selection against the functional disruptions of amino acid variation. Based on this assertion it has been hypothesized that as nsSNPs are more likely to have functional consequences, association studies based on nsSNPs represent a powerful strategy for directly identifying disease-causing associations (Botstein and Risch, 2003).

Adjacent SNPs in the same chromosomal region are not inherited randomly; instead they can be strongly correlated so that entire sets of alleles are inherited together in a haplotype, with an individual receiving one haplotype from each parent. This correlation between alleles is termed linkage disequilibrium (LD), and the strength of LD between two adjacent polymorphisms is dependent on (although not perfectly correlated with) the physical distance between them along the chromosome. Most chromosomal regions are characterized by having a restricted number of common haplotypes which account for much of the genetic variation within any given population. Hence while a chromosomal region may contain many SNP loci, evaluating a few 'tag' SNPs will provide a means of capturing the majority of the genetic variation in the region.

The International HapMap Project (The International HapMap Consortium, 2003) was established to identify and catalogue genetic similarities and differences in humans from different populations. The data generated from this major worldwide initiative provide an invaluable resource for association studies. To date, 270 individuals from four populations: Utah residents with European ancestry, Yoruba from Ibadan in Nigeria, Han Chinese from Beijing and Japanese from Tokyo, have been genotyped for over 3 million SNPs, providing detailed information on the allelic architecture and LD patterns of these ethnic groups.

While there are a number of means of quantifying the strength of LD between a pair of SNPs, r^2 is perhaps the most useful metric in the context of association studies. This is simply defined as the square of the correlation coefficient between the two SNPs in question:

$$\frac{(P_{WM} - P_{W.}P_{.M})^2}{P_{W.}(1 - P_{W.})P_{.M}(1 - P_{.M})} \tag{1.1}$$

where P_{WM} is the probability of the haplotype formed by allele W at SNP 1 and allele M at SNP 2, $P_{W.}$ is the marginal probability of allele W at SNP 1, $P_{.M}$ is the marginal probability of allele M at SNP 2.

Calculation of r^2 is therefore based on the frequencies of the four possible haplotypes of alleles for the two SNPs. In order to calculate these frequencies, the phase of the haplotypes for each individual must either be known or inferred, that is which alleles were co-inherited from each parent. If the genotypes of both parents are known, then unambiguous phased haplotypes of offspring can be generated. However, if such parental information is not available, then phase must be inferred. For some combinations of genotypes, the phase can be inferred with probability 1, for example, if an individual has genotype WW at SNP 1 and genotype MM at SNP 2, then the only possible haplotypes for the individual are two copies of the WM haplotype, one inherited from each parent. However, if the individual is heterozygous at one or more of the SNPs, haplotype phase is unknown. Phased haplotypes for each individual may be inferred using either an expectation-maximization (EM) algorithm or a Markov chain Monte Carlo (MCMC) algorithm and hence haplotype frequencies estimated. Implementations of these algorithms are accessible in a number of publicly available programs, such as Haploview (Barrett *et al.*, 2005) and PHASE (Stephens *et al.*, 2001).

1.3 Direct and indirect association studies

Association studies fall broadly into two main types: direct or sequence-based and indirect or haplotype-based. In a direct association study, the markers genotyped are those which are expected or thought likely to be directly causal of a change in disease risk. Common targets for this kind of approach are markers which are more likely to have functional consequences such as nsSNPs (Smyth *et al.*, 2006) or insertion/deletion polymorphisms. For some of these polymorphisms, direct functional data has been generated. If such data is lacking, missense changes can be analysed according to the biochemical severity of the amino acid substitution and its context within the protein sequence. In the simplest articulation of this, the Grantham matrix (Grantham, 1974) predicts the effect of substitutions between amino acids based on chemical properties, including polarity and molecular volume. More sophisticated *in silico* algorithms have recently been developed which predict the effect of amino acid substitutions on protein structure and activity. Polymorphism Phenotyping (PolyPhen; Ramensky *et al.* 2002) predicts the functional effect of substitutions by assessing the level of sequence conservation between homologous genes over evolutionary time, the physiochemical properties of the exchanged residue and the proximity of the substitution to predicted functional domains and structural features within the protein. Sorting Intolerant from Tolerant (SIFT; Ng and Henikoff 2001) predicts the functional importance of an amino acid substitution based on the alignment of highly similar orthologous and/or paralogous protein sequences. Such algorithms in combination with other considerations such as gene ontology can thus be used to prioritize genotyping efforts (Rudd et al., 2006a; Rudd et al., 2006b; Webb et al., 2006).

The indirect approach makes use of the LD structure of the human genome. In such an approach the markers genotyped are not necessarily thought to have a direct impact on disease risk, associations being a consequence of LD with disease-causing variants. This approach is unbiased and does not depend upon prior knowledge of function or presumptive involvement of any gene in disease causation. This strategy has only recently become feasible for large-scale studies with data generated by HapMap which allow tagging SNPs to be selected that capture a large proportion of the common sequence variation in the human genome.

Recent advances in technology now make it possible to simultaneously score vast numbers of SNPs cost-effectively so that GWAS are now feasible. In a GWAS, typically hundreds of thousands of tag SNPs are genotyped and the aim is to capture as much of the common genetic variation throughout the human genome as possible. Current commercially available platforms allow for the simultaneous genotyping of between 300,000 and 1000,000 SNPs capturing >80% of the common genetic variation in the genome.

An alternative approach to this is the candidate gene approach, where specific genes or pathways are selected for investigation. For example, the established relationship between risk of meningioma and exposure to ionizing radiation provided the rationale for examining whether variants in DNA repair genes contribute to disease susceptibility. Adopting this strategy, Bethke et al. (2008) showed that variation in the DNA repair gene *BRIP1* is associated with risk of meningioma. Candidate gene studies can be undertaken using either the direct or indirect approach. If a direct approach is undertaken, specific markers would be targeted within the genes of interest, whereas in an indirect approach, tagging SNPs would be genotyped in an attempt to capture all the common variation in the selected genes.

1.4 Preliminary analysis and quality control

A number of measures should be implemented to assess data quality before conducting analyses searching for associations with disease risk.

1.4.1 *Assessment of call rates*

The assay performance for some SNPs using any genotyping platform is likely to be suboptimal and may lead to erroneous assignment of genotypes. Two quality metrics relating to call rates are the sample call rate, defined as the number of SNPs that successfully genotyped for each sample; and the SNP call rate, defined as the number of samples for which each SNP was successfully genotyped. Low SNP call rates may indicate that the clustering algorithm used to identify the three possible genotypes is not working optimally and such SNPs should be excluded. Typically call rates of less than 95% are treated cautiously. Differential sample call rates between cases and controls or between batches or plates are indicative of a consistent genotyping problem generating systematic bias.

1.4.2 Duplicate samples

Inclusion of duplicate samples in genotyping assays provides an important means of assessing the performance of the analytical platform, with respect to detecting both within and between batch variations. Ideally genotyping should be undertaken blinded to the inclusion of duplicate samples. The genotypes for each pair of individuals should be compared to determine if DNA from any individual has mistakenly been included multiple times, and any such copies removed. Finally a proportion of genotypes should be checked by subjecting 5% of samples to genotyping on an alternative platform or by directly re-sequencing.

1.4.3 Relatedness between study subjects

Cryptic relatedness between study subjects can be a source of systematic bias. Relatedness between individuals can be determined by calculating inherited-by-state (IBS) sharing probabilities of genotyped SNPs between each pair of study subjects; for each SNP, genotypes for each pair of individuals are compared and assigned a value of 0, 1 or 2 depending on the number of identical alleles. Summing these values over all genotyped SNPs yields a probability distribution for IBS shared values of 0, 1 and 2. A low frequency of IBS = 0 and/or a high percentage of allele sharing (typically >80%) is highly indicative of relatedness and it is prudent to remove one of the subjects from the analysis to reduce bias.

1.4.4 Hardy–Weinberg equilibrium

In a large, randomly mating population, in which there is no migration, or selection against a specific genotype and the mutation rate remains constant, the genotype proportions at a polymorphic variant will be stable from one generation to another, i.e. in Hardy–Weinberg equilibrium (HWE). For a two-allele model where p and $q = 1 - p$ are the allelic frequencies for alleles W and M, respectively, the genotypic frequencies for genotypes WW, WM and MM should be p^2, $2pq$, and q^2, respectively.

Testing for deviation from HWE can be carried out using a χ^2 goodness-of-fit test with one degree of freedom. Low genotype counts can however lead to inflated type I error rates and under these circumstances Fisher's exact test provides a more appropriate test statistic. Provided the controls are in HWE, the cases may also be tested. If a SNP is truly associated with disease risk, then unless this association is mediated in a multiplicative manner, cases will not be in HWE. Hence violation of HWE amongst cases only could indicate the presence of an association with disease risk.

Deviation from HWE in controls can indicate genotyping errors, non-Mendelian inheritance of the SNP in question, inbreeding or population stratification. SNPs showing extreme deviation from HWE in controls should be excluded from further analysis as any association statistics calculated will be hard

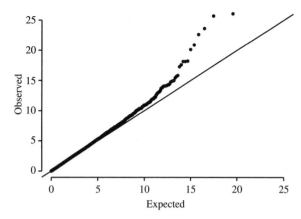

FIG. 1.2: Quantile–quantile (QQ) plot. Under the null hypothesis of Hardy–Weinberg equilibrium, the points are expected to lie on the line $y = x$. The inflation from $y = x$ in the upper tail of the distribution indicates a number of SNPs violating Hardy–Weinberg equilibrium.

to interpret. The question of what constitutes extreme deviation is debatable, but most researchers implement a fairly pragmatic non-conservative cutpoint by adjusting for the number of tests performed using a simple Bonferonni correction, with cutoffs in the range of 10^{-7} for a GWAS.

1.4.5 *Quantile–quantile plots*

Quantile–quantile (QQ) plots provide a useful tool for visualizing the distribution of HWE results and later, the distribution of association statistics. A QQ plot is constructed by plotting the observed ordered test statistics against the test statistics expected under the null hypothesis for a χ^2 distribution with appropriate degrees of freedom (one degree of freedom for the HWE test). Under the null hypothesis of HWE, the plotted points would be expected to lie on the line $y = x$. Systematic inflation from this line indicates a greater number of significant deviations from HWE than expected and could be a consequence of genotyping problems or population stratification (Fig. 1.2).

1.5 Techniques for detecting association

1.5.1 *Single locus tests*

Current strategies for the analysis of the data generated by an association study generally encompass statistical testing carried out on a marker-by-marker basis initially.

For each SNP, genotype data can be represented by the 3×2 table of case-control status against genotype (Table 1.1). Let r_0, r_1, r_2 correspond to the genotype counts for cases and s_0, s_1, s_2 correspond to the genotype counts for controls (Table 1.1a). The most straightforward test of association is provided

TABLE 1.1. Contingency tables showing (a) genotype counts for a single SNP, (b) the dominant test, (c) the recessive test and (d) the allelic test, assuming M is the risk allele.

(a)

	WW	WM	MM	Total
Case	r_0	r_1	r_2	R
Control	s_0	s_1	s_2	S
Total	n_0	n_1	n_2	N

(b)

	WW	WM + MM	Total
Case	r_0	$r_1 + r_2$	R
Control	s_0	$s_1 + s_2$	S
Total	n_0	$n_1 + n_2$	N

(c)

	WW + WM	MM	Total
Case	$r_0 + r_1$	r_2	R
Control	$s_0 + s_1$	s_2	S
Total	$n_0 + n_1$	n_2	N

(d)

	W	M	Total
Case	$2r_0 + r_1$	$r_1 + 2r_2$	R
Control	$2s_0 + s_1$	$s_1 + 2s_2$	S
Total	$2n_0 + n_1$	$n_1 + 2n_2$	N

by the χ^2 test with two degrees of freedom, calculating expected cell counts from the marginal row and column totals in the usual manner. If cell counts are small, i.e. <5, then Fisher's exact test is more appropriate.

The two degree of freedom test statistic may not necessarily be the most powerful test for association as power is dependent on the true nature of the disease model underlying an association. For example, if a SNP impacts on disease risk in a dominant manner, then the most suitable test for detecting the association is calculated from the 2×2 table of case-control status against the two categories formed by pooling rare homozygotes and heterozygotes and comparing against common homozygotes (Table 1.1b). Conversely, if the true model underlying an association is recessive, then the most powerful test for detecting the association is calculated from the 2 × 2 table of case/control status against genotype with common homozygotes and heterozygotes pooled (Table 1.1c). However, since the mode of inheritance is unknown, these tests are not generally utilized as the primary test statistic.

For complex diseases, many biologists believe that either an additive or multiplicative disease model is most likely. Under an additive model, if the heterozygous genotype confers disease risk r, then the rare homozygous genotype confers disease risk $2r$. The Armitage trend test is the most powerful test for association in this scenario and tests the null hypothesis of zero slope for the line fitted to the three genotypic risks. It is defined by:

$$\frac{N(N(r_1 + 2r_2) - R(n_1 + 2n_2))^2}{R(N-R)[N(n_1 + 4n_2) - (n_1 + 2n_2)^2]}. \qquad (1.2)$$

Under a multiplicative model, if the heterozygous genotype confers disease risk r, then the rare homozygous genotype confers disease risk r^2. Genotypes inherited under such a model are most powerfully detected by the allelic test, which is performed by counting the number of W and M alleles amongst cases and controls and then calculating the χ^2 statistic with one degree of freedom from the resulting 2×2 table (or Fisher's exact test if cell counts are small), Table 1.1(d). However, if a multiplicative model does not hold, then HWE is violated in cases and the allele test statistic is invalid (Sasieni, 1997). Instead, the Armitage test for trend is then preferred (note that when HWE holds the Armitage and allele tests are equivalent).

Since there is no single optimum test for all possible genetic models, a compromise is to calculate the test statistic for each SNP as the maximum statistic under dominant, recessive and additive models (Webb et al., 2006). This test statistic is not quite as powerful as if the most efficient test were used, but when the mode of action is not known this loss of power is offset by the reduction in multiple testing. This statistic may be used to rank SNPs, however since its distribution is non-standard, P-values must be calculated empirically.

A QQ plot may be used to visualize association test statistics. Under the null hypothesis of no association, the points would be expected to lie on the line $y = x$; consistent inflation from this line could indicate systematic sources of spurious association (Fig. 1.2).

1.5.2 Incorporating covariates

Some SNPs will affect the risk of cancer more strongly in the presence of other genes or environmental influences. An example of such a gene–environment interaction is provided by the common C677T variant in methylenetetrahydrofolate reductase (*MTHFR*), which leads to disturbed folate metabolism and has been reported to be associated with risks of various common cancers, possibly through either aberrant DNA methylation or availability of nucleotide precursors for DNA synthesis. Perhaps not surprisingly, the effect of *MTHFR* C677T has been reported to be substantially greater in those with lower circulating levels of folate (Ma et al., 1997; Chen et al., 1996).

For a given sample size, strength of interaction and allele frequency, the gain in power achieved by allowing for the interaction depends on the magnitude of the exposure frequency. If such covariate information is available, then association statistics may be calculated adjusting for covariates by logistic regression. It is possible to implement equivalents of each statistical test described above simply by imposing appropriate constraints on the way genotypes are coded in the model. Under the logistic regression model, the binary outcome variable (case-control status) is related to the explanatory variables (SNP genotype plus any other covariates) via the logistic transformation:

$$\ln\left(\frac{p_i}{1-p_i}\right) = \beta_0 X_0 + \beta_1 X_1 + \beta_2 X_2 + \cdots + \beta_p X_p \quad (1.3)$$

where p_i is the risk of cancer for the ith individual, X_0, X_1, X_2 are indicator variables for genotypes WW, WM, MM, respectively (i.e. X_0 is 1 if individual i has genotype WW and 0 otherwise), $X_3, \ldots, X_p$ represent other explanatory variables, and $\beta_0, \ldots, \beta_p$ are the coefficients to be estimated. The most general model which, for large sample sizes is equivalent to the genotypic two degree of freedom test, is obtained by imposing no constraints on β_0, β_1 and β_2. To implement the equivalent of the Armitage test for trend, the constraint $\beta_0 < \beta_1 < \beta_2$ with $\beta_2 - \beta_1 = \beta_1 - \beta_0$ should be applied. For the dominant test $\beta_1 = \beta_2$, and for the recessive test $\beta_1 = \beta_0$. The association statistic for the SNP is then calculated by a likelihood ratio test between the model including the SNP and all other covariates as predictors and the model including all other covariates only as predictors.

Logistic regression is therefore a useful tool if any covariates are thought to impact on case-control status; however the full power of logistic regression comes into force when searching for associations between multiple SNPs and disease risk; this is discussed further below.

1.5.3 Multi-locus tests

Although the SNP-by-SNP analysis approach is the most straightforward to implement, by its very nature it does not utilize information on the relationship between SNPs. One common technique of making use of this information is to exploit the LD structure of the genome to group SNPs in high LD into haplotype blocks. A single statistical test may then be applied to each haplotype block. This can substantially reduce the number of statistical tests undertaken and hence the multiple testing burden, so that power is increased. For each haplotype block if there are k observed haplotypes, the data can be represented by a $2 \times k$ table of case/control status against haplotype. The most straightforward test for association is then the χ^2 test with $k-1$ degrees of freedom, testing the null hypothesis of no difference in haplotype frequencies in cases and controls. One problem with this approach is that since the phase of the genotypes is very rarely known haplotypes themselves must be inferred; loss of power is small as long as LD is near-perfect; if LD is weaker, then this approach is not advisable.

An issue with this type of approach is the question of how information about similarity between haplotypes should be incorporated into a model. For example if two haplotypes differ by only one allele, they are more likely to have a comparable impact on disease risk than a haplotype where many alleles differ. One means of addressing this is to integrate this information into the analysis by using a clustering approach to group together sets of haplotypes that are likely to share recent common ancestry (i.e. with fewer mutation events separating them). The subsequent statistical test would have fewer degrees of freedom but could again suffer from loss of power if there is a reasonable amount of uncertainty about the relationship between haplotypes.

The haplotype-based analysis approach is therefore most useful when LD blocks and hence haplotypes are clearly defined and well-delineated, a situation more likely to occur if the density of SNP genotyping is high. It perhaps has less utility if a tagging approach has been used to select SNPs for genotyping as tag SNPs by their very definition will not constitute extensive blocks of strong LD.

1.5.4 Interactive and additive effects

The 'common-disease common-variant' model of cancer susceptibility implies that variation in disease risk will be a consequence of interactions between different genetic variants and also between genetic and environmental factors, acting either additively or multiplicatively. Under this assumption, an alternative analysis approach which systematically fits models allowing for interactions between loci has been shown to have greater power to identify risk variants (Marchini et al., 2005) even when accounting for the increased multiple testing burden. The approach utilizes logistic regression to fit each pair of SNPs and their interaction concurrently. However, when the single-locus effects are large relative to the interaction effects, this approach does not provide any improvement in power over the SNP-by-SNP approach. A compromise between the two approaches could be to first identify a set of associated single loci under liberal statistical criteria and then evaluate all possible two-way interactions among them under rigorous criteria, corrected for multiple testing.

If data are available on environmental factors then it is also possible to search for gene–environment interactive effects by including the environmental variable with the SNP in a logistic regression model. A more efficient approach to detecting this kind of epistasis is to conduct a case-only regression analysis where the response is the variable hypothesised to interact with the genetic variant, which is itself fitted as an explanatory variable. A case-only analysis provides increased power to detect gene–environment interactions than a case-control analysis based on the same number of cases (Yang et al., 1997).

An important feature of the polygenic model is that most susceptible individuals are at elevated risk because of the combined effects of several susceptibility alleles; as multiple risk loci are identified, the combined effects of these may be examined, whether interactive or additive. For example, Tomlinson et al. (2008) examined the combined risk of the five low penetrance alleles identified thus far for colorectal cancer. There was no evidence of interactive effects between any of these SNPs; however assigning two for a variant homozygote and one for a heterozygote, the risk of colorectal cancer increased significantly with increasing numbers of variant alleles for the five loci, with individuals carrying seven or more deleterious alleles being at $\sim$ three-fold increased risk of colorectal cancer. Based on these data, the five SNPs identified thus far have potential to be clinically useful.

1.5.5 Pathway analysis

The 'common-disease common-variant' hypothesis implies that it is unlikely that any one single genetic polymorphism would have a dramatic effect on cancer risk. A pathway-based genotyping approach, which assesses the combined effects of a panel of polymorphisms that interact in the same pre-defined biological pathway, may amplify the effects of individual polymorphisms and enhance the predictive power. The standard analysis method is to then count the number of 'risk' alleles that each individual carries and compare the distribution of this random variable in cases and controls, using logistic regression to adjust for other covariates. To search for higher-order gene–gene interactions, classification and regression tree (CART) analysis may be perfomed. This is a binary recursive-partitioning method that produces a decision tree to identify subgroups of subjects at higher risk. The algorithm, as implemented in HelixTree Software, uses inference-based recursive modelling to determine the SNP (or other risk factor) at which the first locally optimal split of subjects occurs. The process continues with multiplicity-adjusted P-values to control tree growth, until the subject subgroups have no subsequent statistically significant splits or reach a prespecified minimum size. This approach has been successfully applied to genes in the DNA repair and cell cycle control pathways for bladder cancer (Wu et al., 2006).

1.5.6 Subgroup analysis

Another biological hypothesis is that the impact of a genetic variant on disease risk may be variable dependent on an individual's phenotype. This is particularly probable for a complex disease such as cancer where the phenotype can be classified into distinct groups. For example colorectal cancers can be classified into microsatellite stable (MSS) and microsatellite instable (MSI) cancers and the effect of the C677T variant in *MTHFR* varies according to MS status. A recent study showed that when *MTHFR* C677T genotype frequencies in MSS colorectal cancer cases were compared to controls, individuals with homozygous variant genotype were at 19% reduced risk of cancer compared to wild type. Conversely, when MSI colorectal cancer cases were compared to controls, individuals with one or two *MTHFR* 677T alleles were at 42% increased cancer risk (Hubner et al., 2007). These observations indicate that *MTHFR* 677TT homozygous individuals are more likely to develop MSI colorectal cancer than those with wild type genotype, and this common polymorphism has differential influences on MSI and MSS colorectal cancer risk.

In addition to standard case-control analysis methods restricted to the subgroup in question, this hypothesis may also be assessed using the case-only regression analysis described above. When conducting a subgroup analysis, it is important that phenotypes defining subgroups be well defined and have strong biological basis. Otherwise the temptation could be to continue defining subgroups in post-hoc analyses until a statistically significant association is identified, however meaningless.

1.5.7 Imputation of genotypes

Currently, association studies are based on genotyping a proportion of the known SNPs in the human genome and the cost of sequencing the entire genome for large numbers of individuals is prohibitive. However it is possible to use data from the HapMap, estimates of the fine-scale recombination map across the genome and a population genetic model to accurately infer genotypes for SNPs not directly assayed in the study (Marchini et al., 2007). Inference of genotypes allows for finer mapping of regions of interest and also has utility for validation and correction of data at genotyped markers. Furthermore, imputation of genotypes at markers not directly assayed also provides the possibility of combining data from multiple genome-wide scans that have used different SNP sets, since all SNPs genotyped in any of the studies may be inferred in other studies. By extensively increasing the number of individuals for whom genotype information is available, such a strategy has the potential to provide a considerable increase in power to detect associations with cancer risk.

1.5.8 Confounding and stratification

Population stratification, where cases and controls disproportionately represent regionally or ethnically defined genetic subgroups, can result in spurious associations between disease and any genetic marker with allele frequencies that differ between the subgroups. The potentially confounding effect of population stratification should in principle be allowed for in the design and analysis of a study. One method of circumventing the problem is to use family-based controls. The most common approach is the transmission disequilibrium test (TDT; Spielman et al. 1994), which assesses the evidence for preferential transmission of one allele over the other from heterozygous parents. For complex late-onset diseases such as cancer, the non-availability of parental genotypes means that the TDT approach is often impractical. Allied statistics based only on sibling genotypes have been devised to obviate the requirement for parental genotypes, but all involve additional genotyping. Moreover, such restrictions on eligibility inevitably lead to smaller studies and these tests are also inherently less powerful than conventional case-control methods (Risch and Teng, 1998). If cases and controls are well matched, differences in the frequency of genotypes will only be seen at predisposition loci. Although population stratification remains a potential problem its effects within large studies have generally been rather exaggerated and can usually be addressed by suitable analysis.

The genomic control approach (Devlin and Roeder, 1999) is most commonly used, where an inflation factor λ is calculated by comparing the median of the observed Armitage trend test statistics with the median of the expected distribution (χ^2 with one degree of freedom). A value of $\lambda > 1$ represents an inflation of the test statistics from those expected by chance which is a likely consequence of population stratification. Genomic control normalizes test statistics by dividing by λ so that the resulting test statistics represent associations after adjustment for population stratification.

If the subgroups causing the inflation can be accurately identified, for example, by ascertaining the region of origin for each individual, then it is possible to stratify for them in the analysis. If such classification data are not available, clustering approaches such as those implemented in the STRUCTURE (Pritchard et al., 2000) and EIGENSTRAT (Price et al., 2006) programs, may be used to group individuals on the basis of the genotype data alone. This information can then be incorporated into the analysis; however it is not always clear what the groupings actually represent.

1.6 Statistical power and multiple testing

The last 10 years have seen a dramatic rise in the number of published studies reporting the relationship between SNPs in candidate genes and the risk of cancer. Despite this considerable effort, however, few disease loci have been identified unequivocally. Published systematic reviews on specific polymorphisms and risk of breast (Dunning et al., 1999) and colorectal (Houlston and Tomlinson, 2001) cancer illustrate this apparent failure. In a review of 50 studies of the effects of common alleles of 13 genes on risk of colorectal cancer 16 significant associations ($P < 0.05$) were seen, but only three were reported in more than one study and there were only three significant associations in the pooled data (for *APC*-I1307K, *HRAS1*-VNTR and *MTHFR*Val/Val). A systematic review of 46 studies on the effects on breast cancer risk of 18 different genes revealed 12 statistically significant associations. None was reported in more than one study, and the pooled analysis gave a significant difference in genotype frequency for only three SNPs (*CYP19*-(TTTA)10, *GSTP1*-Ile105Val and *TP53*-Arg72Pro). These results illustrate the dangers of imposing too lenient a significance threshold for declaring a positive association. For many of these candidate genes, there was little prior evidence of involvement of the specific locus and the associated *P*-values should in principle be adjusted by Bayesian methods, using prior probabilities based on the strength of the evidence that they are involved in cancer aetiology or that the specific type of germline variation affects the structure or level of the expressed protein.

The appropriate threshold for defining statistical significance in any association study is an important consideration. As the number of possible risk alleles is very large, the prior probability that any random SNP tested will be associated with disease susceptibility will be low. If a significance level of 5% is used to define a significant result, then by definition the corresponding type I error rate (i.e. the probability of an association being declared true when it is, in fact, false) is 5%. Consequently, if 500,000 SNPs are to be tested on a loci-by-loci basis, 25,000 SNPs will display nominally significant associations purely by chance. Amongst those results, it is expected that there will reside a subset of SNPs where the association is truly causal. The simplest response to the multiple testing issue is to employ a Bonferroni correction, dividing the global significance level by the number of tests undertaken. For a GWAS, this leads to a required individual test P-value to the order of 10^{-7} to declare a significant result. The Bonferroni correction is however overly stringent if the markers tested are not independent, as is likely to be the case in a GWAS.

An alternative approach to controlling the type I error rate is to instead control the false discovery rate (FDR), that is, the proportion of false positive associations among all positives (Benjamini and Hochberg, 1995). This leads to a global threshold that is adaptive to the data. That is, if a higher percentage of the null hypotheses tested are truly false, the FDR procedure will identify a lower cutoff level than the universal Bonferroni cutoff, therefore improving power.

An empirical approach to the multiple testing problem is to conduct a permutation procedure. This is an iterative approach that samples from the null hypothesis of no association between SNP and case-control status so that empirical P-values can be generated. At each iteration, the case-control labels are permuted and then the association statistics re-calculated. By permuting the case/control labels, any true associations between SNP and disease risk are nullified so that the association statistics calculated at each iteration represent samples from the null hypothesis, taking into account the complex correlation structure between genotyped SNPs. The true association statistics are then compared with this null distribution to generate empirical P-values. Permutation procedures are extremely computationally intensive and time consuming. One way of speeding up these procedures is to generate a smaller number of permutations than would usually be required and then fit an extreme value distribution to the observed maximum statistics (Dudbridge and Koeleman, 2004). Further permutations are then generated to tune the parameters of the fitted distribution.

Consideration of sample size is clearly essential in the design of association studies because of the issues of generating true- and false-positive results and replicating findings. The sample sizes required depend upon SNP allele frequency, the magnitude of the effect, and the power and significance level stipulated for defining a positive test.

Segregation analyses and recent results from GWAS of colorectal, breast and prostate cancers suggest that genetic variants impacting on cancer risk will confer relative risks of 1.1–1.5 in carriers. In order for an association study to have reasonable power to detect effects of this size at the small significance levels required, large collections of cases and controls are essential. Figure 1.3 shows the sample size requirements to detect an association at the 10^{-4} significance level with power of 80% by relative risk and allele frequency, assuming equal numbers of cases and controls. For a SNP with 20% minor allele frequency

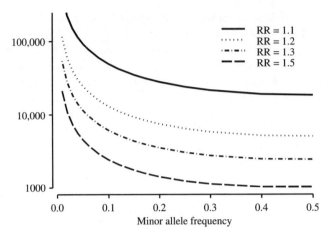

FIG. 1.3: Sample sizes required to detect an association at 10^{-4} level with power of 80% by minor allele frequency and relative risk.

conferring a per-allele increase of 1.3 in cancer risk, ∼3500 cases and controls would be required to detect an association. Clearly studies based on less than 1000 cases and 1000 controls will rarely have adequate power to detect even the most common variants associated with cancer risk.

1.6.1 Design strategies for increasing power

Analysis of unselected cases is satisfactory for the evaluation of common alleles but has limited power if the carrier frequency is less than 5%. Restricting the study to early-onset cases or pathologically defined subsets might increase the power, but in the absence of good evidence for a different genetic basis in younger patients or in those with a particular histology such restrictions on eligibility may merely reduce the available sample size. The power of association studies can, however, be significantly enhanced by cases selected for a family history of cancer. Houlston and Peto (2003) and Antoniou and Easton (2003) calculated the power of association studies based on unselected and familial cases. Assuming two controls per case, a dominant allele conferring a relative risk of 2.0 carried by 5% of the population would be detectable using 800 unselected cases. If the prevalence were only 1% in controls, however, 3700 unselected cases would be required. In contrast, if the cases analysed had two affected relatives the number required would be reduced from 3700 to 700, a more than five-fold reduction in laboratory costs. Bilateral breast cancer patients should prove particularly informative in this respect. They can be identified systematically through cancer registries, yet they are as powerful as cases with two affected relatives.

The potential of association studies of familial cases to detect rare susceptibility alleles conferring a relative risk of less than 2.0 is illustrated by the *CHEK2* 1100delC mutation in breast cancer patients. This allele, which is carried by 1% of the population, confers a 1.7-fold increase in breast cancer risk (Meijers-Heijboer et al., 2002). The prevalence was not significantly increased among unselected breast cancer cases (1.4%), but was greatly increased among familial cases not carrying *BRCA1* or *BRCA2* mutations (5.1%; $P < 10^{-7}$). The relative risk in pooled data on unselected cases was 2.3 (CHEK2 Breast Cancer Case-Control Consortium, 2004).

1.6.2 The staged design

A staged association study design provides a means of offsetting some of the costs of conducting a GWAS. In this design, all SNPs are genotyped in a subset of the cases and controls. Those SNPS most significantly associated with risk, typically at the 5% level are genotyped in the remaining cases and controls. The strategy minimizes the amount of genotyping required and hence reduces the cost of the project whilst retaining a high power to identify SNPs associated with a modest risk. Although the power of the staged design will never exceed the power of a single stage design if the same number of cases and controls are available, it is possible by choosing the proportions of samples and SNPs genotyped in each stage appropriately to attain almost equal power to the single-stage approach. Genotyping genetically enriched cases in the first stage provides a highly efficient strategy for achieving the best power-to-genotyping ratio.

1.7 Replication, quantification, and identification of causal variants

Once an association has been detected in the initial study population, it is highly desirable to replicate this observation in further independent study populations. This is useful for two reasons: firstly it provides robust evidence of the association and negates the possibility that the observed association is due to confounding factors such as extreme population stratification or differential genotyping problems. Secondly, it can offer valuable information on the nature of the association and be used to provide more robust estimates of disease risk. For example, knowledge of the risk model could provide insight into the biological mechanisms underlying the association. Further subgroup analysis at this stage could also be useful to provide insight into the aetiology of the observed association.

After replication of an observed association, the challenge of identifying the causal locus still remains. A sequence-based association study directly targeting SNPs with a high prior probability of functionality implies higher probability that the causal variant has been directly genotyped; however the possibility of the observed association being a consequence of LD still remains. Therefore all genetic variants lying within the limits of the region of association must be thoroughly interrogated.

Before conducting any further experimental work, various techniques may be used to refine the region of association. One such approach is to consider genealogical trees in the form of ancestral recombination graphs (ARGs) that could explain the recombination and mutation event history in the individuals in the study (Minichiello and Durbin, 2006). For each tree generated, the branches of the tree are examined for clustering of disease cases which would suggest that a causative mutation occurred on that branch. Probabilities are then averaged over all trees. This approach has been shown to give increased accuracy in positioning causative loci.

In order to further refine the region of association, samples from different ethnic groups may be of utility. If the association with disease risk is replicated in a cohort with different ethnic background, the LD structure of the new population can be interrogated to further refine the region. Populations with higher rates of recombination such as those with African origins may be particularly useful. Variants in the *SMAD7* gene have recently been shown to be associated with colorectal cancer risk in the European population (Broderick et al., 2007). Figure 1.4 shows the LD patterns in CEPH and Chinese populations from HapMap for the *SMAD7* locus. Since the LD patterns in the region are quite different, a case-control analysis based on individuals from the Chinese population should help to further refine the association region. Further genotyping efforts may focus on those variants which lie in coding regions or areas of high conservation.

Final evidence for causality of any variant mapping to the associated region may ultimately be contingent on functional assays. However such work will inevitably be predicated on robust statistical evidence for a true association.

1.8 Discussion

Around 30 years ago, Anderson (1974) stated that the 2/3-fold excess risk seen in first-degree relatives of cancer patients 'is not indicative of strong genetic effects. They are more suggestive of the involvement of many genes with small effects acting in concert with environmental or nongenetic factors with larger and more important effects'. This was a statistical fallacy (Peto, 1980), but paradoxically there is growing evidence from GWAS of breast, colorectal and prostate cancer that the conclusion is correct for these malignancies and perhaps for many other common cancers. Although the risks associated with each allele may be individually modest, they are likely in combination to contribute a substantial proportion of overall cancer incidence, and considerably more than the high-penetrance genes so far identified.

In the future, association studies are likely to play an increasing role in the search for novel cancer susceptibility genes. After years of poorly powered association studies generating mainly type I errors, recent advances in technology have heralded the advent of association studies based on large numbers of samples, often genotyped over many SNPs. The robust statistical techniques described in this chapter are available to analyse the data generated from association studies, and the recent discovery of many novel low penetrance cancer susceptibility loci demonstrates the success of this study design.

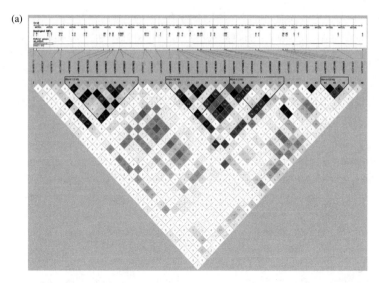

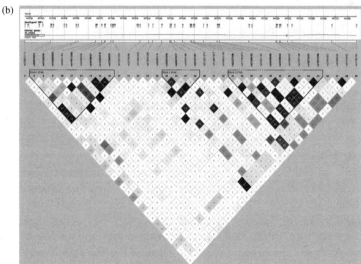

FIG. 1.4: Linkage disequilibrium patterns in (a) CEPH and (b) Chinese populations for the *SMAD7* locus associated with colorectal cancer risk. Dark squares indicate strong linkage disequilibrium while light squares indicate weak linkage disequilibrium.

1.9 URLs

- HapMap: http://www.hapmap.org
- Haploview: http://www.broad.mit.edu/mpg/haploview/
- R: http://www.r-project.org/

- Phase: http://stephenslab.uchicago.edu/software.html
- Impute: http://www.stats.ox.ac.uk/marchini/software/gwas/impute.html
- Structure: http://pritch.bsd.uchicago.edu/structure.html
- Eigenstrat: http://genepath.med.harvard.edu/reich/Software.htm
- HelixTree: http://www.goldenhelix.com/SNP_Variation/HelixTree/helixtree.html

References

Amundadottir, L. T., Sulem, P., Gudmundsson, J., Helgason, A., Baker, A., Agnarsson, B. A., Sigurdsson, A., Benediktsdottir, K. R., Cazier, J. B., Sainz, J., Jakobsdottir, M., Kostic, J., Magnusdottir, D. N., Ghosh, S., Agnarsson, K., Birgisdottir, B., Roux, L. Le, Olafsdottir, A., Blondal, T., Andresdottir, M., Gretarsdottir, O. S., Bergthorsson, J. T., Gudbjartsson, D., Gylfason, A., Thorleifsson, G., Manolescu, A., Kristjansson, K., Geirsson, G., Isaksson, H., Douglas, J., Johansson, J. E., Bälter, K., Wiklund, F., Montie, J. E., Yu, X., Suarez, B. K., Ober, C., Cooney, K. A., Gronberg, H., Catalona, W. J., Einarsson, G. V., Barkardottir, R. B., Gulcher, J. R., Kong, A., Thorsteinsdottir, U., and Stefansson, K. (2006). A common variant associated with prostate cancer in european and african populations. *Nature Genetics*, **38**, 652–8.

Anderson, D. E. (1974). Genetic study of breast cancer: identification of a high risk group. *Cancer*, **34**, 1090–7.

Anglian Breast Cancer Study Group (2000). Prevalence and penetrance of *BRCA1* and *BRCA2* mutations in a population-based series of breast cancer cases. *British Journal of Cancer*, **83**, 1301–8.

Antoniou, A. C. and Easton, D. F. (2003). Polygenic inheritance of breast cancer: Implications for design of association studies. *Genetic Epidemiology*, **25**, 190–202.

Barrett, J. C., Fry, B., Maller, J., and Daly, M. J. (2005). Haploview: analysis and visualization of LD and haplotype maps. *Bioinformatics*, **21**, 263–5.

Benjamini, Y. and Hochberg, Y. (1995). Controlling the false discovery rate: a practical and powerful approach to multiple testing. *Journal of the Royal Statistical Society B*, **57**, 289–300.

Bethke, L., Murray, A., Webb, E., Schoemaker, M., Muir, K., McKinney, P., Hepworth, S., Dimitropoulou, P., Lophatananon, A., Feychting, M., Lonn, S., Ahlborn, A., Malmer, B., Henriksson, R., Auvinen, A., Kiuru, A., Salminen, T., Johansen, C., Christensen, H. Collatz, Kosteljanetz, M., Swerdlow, A., and Houlston, R. (2008). Analysis of DNA repair SNPs identifies a common genetic risk factor for meningioma. *Journal of the National Cancer Institute*, **100**, 270–6.

Bodmer, W. F., Bailey, C. J., Bodmer, J., Bussey, H. J., Ellis, A., Gorman, P., Lucibello, F. C., Murday, V. A., Rider, S. H., Scambler, P., Sheer, D.,

Solomon, E., and Spurr, N. K. (1987). Localization of the gene for familial adenomatous polyposis on chromosome 5. *Nature*, **328**, 614–6.

Botstein, D. and Risch, N. (2003). Discovering genotypes underlying human phenotypes: past successes for mendelian disease, future approaches for complex disease. *Nature Genetics*, **33 Suppl**, 228–37.

Broderick, P., Carvajal-Carmona, L., Pittman, A. M., Webb, E., Howarth, K., Rowan, A., Lubbe, S., Spain, S., Sullivan, K., Fielding, S., Jaeger, E., Vijayakrishnan, J., Kemp, Z., Gorman, M., Chandler, I., Papaemmanuil, E., Penegar, S., Wood, W., Sellick, G., Qureshi, M., Teixeira, A., Domingo, E., Barclay, E., Martin, L., Sieber, O., CORGI Consortium, Kerr, D., Gray, R., Peto, J., Cazier, J. B., Tomlinson, I., and Houlston, R. S. (2007). A genome-wide association study shows that common alleles of smad7 influence colorectal cancer risk. *Nature Genetics*, **39**, 1315–7.

Cannon-Albright, L. A., Goldgar, D. E., Meyer, L. J., Lewis, C. M., Anderson, D. E., Fountain, J. W., Hegi, M. E., Wiseman, R. W., Petty, E. M., Bale A. E., Olopade, O. I, Diaz, M. O., Kwiatkowski, D. J., Piepkorn, M. W, Zone, J. J, and Skolnick, M. H. (1992). Assignment of a locus for familial melanoma, MLM, to chromosome 9p13-p22. *Science*, **258**, 1148–52.

CHEK2 Breast Cancer Case-Control Consortium (2004). Chek2*1100delc and susceptibility to breast cancer: a collaborative analysis involving 10,860 breast cancer cases and 9,065 controls from 10 studies. *American Journal of Human Genetics*, **74**, 1175–82.

Chen, J., Giovannucci, E., Kelsey, K., Rimm, E. B., Stampfer, M. J., Colditz, G. A., Spiegelman, D., Willett, W. C., and Hunter, D. J. (1996). A methylenetetrahydrofolate reductase polymorphism and the risk of colorectal cancer. *Cancer Research*, **56**, 4862–4864.

Devlin, B. and Roeder, K. (1999). Genomic control for association studies. *Biometrics*, **55**, 997–1004.

Dudbridge, F. and Koeleman, B. P. (2004). Efficient computation of significance levels for multiple associations in large studies of correlated data, including genomewide association studies. *American Journal of Human Genetics*, **75**, 424–35.

Dunning, A. M., Healey, C. S., Pharoah, P. D., Teare, M. D., Ponder, B. A., and Easton, D. F. (1999). A systematic review of genetic polymorphisms and breast cancer risk. *Cancer Epidemiology Biomarkers and Prevention*, **8**, 843–54.

Easton, D. F., Pooley, K. A., Dunning, A. M., Pharoah, P. D., Thompson, D., Ballinger, D. G., Struewing, J. P., Morrison, J., and Field, H. (2007). Genome-wide association study identifies novel breast cancer susceptibility loci. *Nature*, **447**, 1087–93.

Grantham, R. (1974). Amino acid difference formula to help explain protein evolution. *Science*, **185**, 862–4.

Hall, J. M., Lee, M. K., Newman, B., Morrow, J. E., Anderson, L. A., Huey, B., and King, M. C. (1990). Linkage of early-onset familial breast cancer to chromosome 17q21. *Science*, **250**, 1684–9.

Houlston, R. S. and Peto, J. (2003). The future of association studies of common cancers. *Human Genetics*, **112**, 434–5.

Houlston, R. S. and Tomlinson, I. P. (2001). Polymorphisms and colorectal tumor risk. *Gastroenterology*, **121**, 282–301.

Hubner, R. A., Lubbe, S., Chandler, I., and Houlston, R. (2007). MTHFR C677T has differential influence on risk of MSI and MSS colorectal cancer. *Human Molecular Genetics*, **16**, 1072–7.

Lichtenstein, P., V., N., Verkasalo, P. K., Iliadou, A., Kaprio, J., Koskenvuo, M., Pukkala, E., Skytthe, A., and Hemminki, K. (2000). Environmental and heritable factors in the causation of cancer-analyses of cohorts of twins from Sweden, Denmark, and Finland. *New England Journal of Medicine*, **343**, 78–85.

Lindblom, A., Tannergrd, P., Werelius, B., and Nordenskjld, M. (1993). Genetic mapping of a second locus predisposing to hereditary non-polyposis colon cancer. *Nature Genetics*, **5**, 279–82.

Marchini, J., Donnelly, P., and Cardon, L. R. (2005). Genome-wide strategies for detecting multiple loci that influence complex diseases. *Nature Genetics*, **37**, 413–7.

Marchini, J., Howie, B., Myers, S., McVean, G., and Donnelly, P. (2007). A new multipoint method for genome-wide association studies by imputation of genotypes. *Nature Genetics*, **39**, 906–13.

Ma, J., Stampfer, M., Giovannucci, E., Artigas, C., Hunter, D., Fuchs, C., Willett, W., Selhub, J., Hennekens, C., and Rozen, R. (1997). Methylenetetrahydrofolate reductase polymorphism, dietary interactions, and risk of colorectal cancer. *Cancer Research*, **57**, 1098–1102.

Meijers-Heijboer, H., van den Ouweland, A., Klijn, J., and Wasielewski, M. (2002). Low-penetrance susceptibility to breast cancer due to CHEK2(*)1100delC in noncarriers of *BRCA1* or *BRCA2* mutations. *Nature Genetics*, **31**, 55–9.

Minichiello, M. J. and Durbin, R. (2006). Mapping trait loci by use of inferred ancestral recombination graphs. *American Journal of Human Genetics*, **79**, 910–22.

Ng, P. C. and Henikoff, S. (2001). Predicting deleterious amino acid substitutions. *Genome Research*, **11**, 863–74.

Peltomaki, P., Aaltonen, L. A., Sistonen, P., and L, L. Pylkknen (1993). Genetic mapping of a locus predisposing to human colorectal cancer. *Science*, **260**, 810–2.

Peto, J. (1980). Genetic predisposition to cancer. In *Banbury Report 4: Cancer Incidence in Defined Populations* (ed. G. J, L. JL, and S. M), pp. 203–213. Cold Spring Harbor, N.Y.: Cold Spring Harbor Laboratory.

Peto, J. (2002). Breast cancer susceptibility-a new look at an old model. *Cancer Cell*, **1**, 411–2.

Pharoah, P. D., Antoniou, A., Bobrow, M., Zimmern, R. L., Easton, D. F., and Ponder, B. A. (2002). Polygenic susceptibility to breast cancer and implications for prevention. *Nature Genetics*, **31**, 33–6.

Price, A. L., Patterson, N. J., Plenge, R. M., Weinblatt, M. E., Shadick, N. A., and Reich, D. (2006). Principal components analysis corrects for stratification in genome-wide association studies. *Nature Genetics*, **38**, 904–9.

Pritchard, J. K., Stephens, M., and Donnelly, P. (2000). Inference of population structure using multilocus genotype data. *Genetics*, **155**, 945–59.

Ramensky, V., Bork, P., and Sunyaev, S. (2002). Human non-synonymous SNPs: server and survey. *Nucleic Acids Research*, **30**, 3894–900.

Risch, N. and Merikangas, K. (1996). The future of genetic studies of complex human diseases. *Science*, **273**, 1516–7.

Risch, N. and Teng, J. (1998). The relative power of family-based and case-control designs for linkage disequilibrium studies of complex human diseases I. DNA pooling. *Genome Research*, **8**, 1273–88.

Rudd, M. F., Sellick, G. S., Webb, E. L., Catovsky, D., and Houlston, R. S. (2006a). Variants in the *atm-brca2-chek2* axis predispose to chronic lymphocytic leukemia. *Blood*, **108**, 638–44.

Rudd, M. F., Webb, E. L., Matakidou, A., Sellick, G. S., Williams, R. D., Bridle, H., Eisen, T., Houlston, R. S., and GELCAPS Consortium (2006b). Variants in the GH-IGF axis confer susceptibility to lung cancer. *Genome Research*, **16**, 693–701.

Sasieni, P. D. (1997). From genotypes to genes: doubling the sample size. *Biometrics*, **53**, 1253–61.

Smyth, D. J., Cooper, J. D., Bailey, R., Field, S., and Burren, C. (2006). A genome-wide association study of nonsynonymous SNPs identifies a type 1 diabetes locus in the interferon-induced helicase (IFIH1) region. *Nature Genetics*, **38**, 617–9.

Spielman, R. S., McGinnis, R. E., and Ewens, W. J. (1994). The transmission/disequilibrium test detects cosegregation and linkage. *American Journal of Human Genetics*, **54**, 559–60.

Stephens, M., Smith, N., and Donnelly, P. (2001). A new statistical method for haplotype reconstruction from population data. *American Journal of Human Genetics*, **68**, 978–989.

The International HapMap Consortium (2003). The International HapMap Project. *Nature*, **426**, 789–796.

Tomlinson, I., Webb, E., Carvajal-Carmona, L., Broderick, P., Kemp, Z., Spain, S., Penegar, S., Chandler, I., Gorman, M., Wood, W., Barclay, E., Lubbe, S., Martin, L., Sellick, G., Jaeger, E., Hubner, R., Wild, R., Rowan, A., Fielding, S., Howarth, K., CORGI Consortium, Silver, A., Atkin, W., Muir, K., Logan, R., Kerr, D., Johnstone, E., Sieber, O., Gray, R., Thomas, H., Peto, J., Cazier, J. B., and Houlston, R. (2007). A genome-wide association scan of tag SNPs identifies a susceptibility variant for colorectal cancer at 8q24.21. *Nature Genetics*, **39**, 984–8.

Tomlinson, I. P. M., Webb, E., Carvajal-Carmona, L., Broderick, P., Howarth, K., Pittman, A. M., Spain, S., Lubbe, S., Walther, A., Sullivan, K., Jaeger, E., Fielding, S., Rowan, A., Vijayakrishnan, J., Domingo, E.,

Chandler, I., Kemp, Z., Qureshia, M., Farrington, S. M., Tenesa, A., Prendergast, J. G. D., Barnetson, R. A., Penegar, S., Barclay, E., Wood, W., Martin, L., Gorman, M., Thomas, H., Peto, J., Bishop, D. T., Gray, R., Maher, E. R., Lucassen, A., Kerr, D., Evans, D. G. R., The CORGI Consortium, Schafmayer, C., Buch, S., Völzke, H., Hampe, J., Schreiber, S., John, U., Koessler, T., Pharoah, P., van Wezel, T., Morreau, H., Wijnen, J. T., Hopper, J. L., Southey, M. C., Giles, G. G., Severi, G., Castellv-Bel, S., Ruiz-Ponte, C., Carracedo, A., Castells, A., The EPICOLON Consortium, Försti, A., Hemminki, K., Vodicka, P., Naccarati, A., Lipton, L., Ho, J. W. C., Cheng, K. K., Sham, P. C., Luk, J., Agúndez, J. A. G., Ladero, J. M., de la Hoya, M., Calds, T., Niittymäki, I., Tu (2008). A genome-wide association study identifies novel colorectal cancer susceptibility loci on chromosomes 10p14 and 8q23.3. *Nature Genetics*, **40**, 623–30.

Webb, E. L., Rudd, M. F., Sellick, G. S., Galta, R. El, Bethke, L., Wood, W., Fletcher, O., Penegar, S., Withey, L., Qureshi, M., Johnson, N., Tomlinson, I., Gray, R., Peto, J., and Houlston, R. S. (2006). Search for low penetrance alleles for colorectal cancer through a scan of 1467 non-synonymous SNPs in 2575 cases and 2707 controls with validation by kin-cohort analysis of 14 704 first-degree relatives. *Human Molecular Genetics*, **15**, 3263–71.

Wooster, R., Neuhausen, S. L., Mangion, J., Quirk, Y., Ford, D., Collins, N., Nguyen, K., Seal, S., Tran, T., Averill, D., Fields, P., Marshall, G., Narod, S., Lenoir, G. M., Lynch, H., Feunteun, J., Devilee, P., Cornelisse, C. J., Menko, F. H., Daly, P. A., Ormiston, W., McManus, R., Pye, C., Lewis, C. M., Cannon–Albright, L.A., Peto, J., Ponder, B. A. J., Skolnick, M. H., Easton, D. F., Goldgar, D. E., Stratton, M. R. (1994). Localization of a breast cancer susceptibility gene, *BRCA2*, to chromosome 13q12-13. *Science*, **265**, 2088–90.

Wu, X., Gu, J., Grossman, H. B., Amos, C. I., Etzel, C., Huang, M., Zhang, Q., Millikan, R. E., Lerner, S., Dinney, C. P., and Spitz, M. R. (2006). Bladder cancer predisposition: a multigenic approach to DNA repair and cell-cycle-control genes. *The American Journal of Human Genetics*, **78**, 464–479.

Yang, Q., Khoury, M. J., and Flanders, W. D. (1997). Sample size requirements in case-only designs to detect gene-environment interaction. *American Journal of Epidemiology*, **146**, 713–720.

2

METHODS FOR DNA COPY NUMBER DERIVATIONS

Cameron Brennan

2.1 Copy number aberration in cancer

Chromosomal copy number aberrations (CNA) are a common form of genomic mutation in cancer. Like point mutations, translocations and epigenetic alterations, CNA may directly contribute to tumour pathogenesis and also may generically reflect genomic instability occurring during tumour evolution. CNA is defined simply as variation from the full chromosomal complement of germline cells: either loss of one or both normal copies or gain of extra copies. A gene which is completely deleted is essentially removed from the cell's transcriptome; a gene amplified by many extra copies is often overexpressed as a result. For molecular profiling in cancer research, CNA data is particularly attractive because genomic amplification and deletion generate immediate hypotheses for their biological impact: many established tumour suppressors are known to be genomically deleted in cancer and many known oncogenes have been discovered by their inclusion in amplifications. It stands to reason that newly characterized focal CNA events could point to novel cancer-relevant genes, micro-RNAs or other functional genomic elements. In contrast, gene expression profiling of a tumour might reveal hundreds or thousands of genes to be differentially expressed compared to normal tissue, often with little further evidence to identify which of these are functionally significant. Expression microarray technology has matured and there are well-developed analytical methods to analyse most forms of expression data. In comparison, there has been a relative lag in the development of high-throughput techniques for ascertaining chromosomal copy number and in the development of methods to analyse this data. The conceptual simplicity of CNA belies the complexity of analysis needed to identify biologically and statistically significant events and to distinguish noise and artifacts. This chapter will introduce some of the major technologies and methods used to generate and analyse copy number data.

2.2 Obtaining and analysing copy number data: platforms and initial processing

Chromosomal copy number can be assayed by a variety of microarray and sequencing methods that will be briefly described here. The methods differ in sensitivity, resolution, cost, and DNA requirement, and some provide allelic or sequence information in addition to copy number.

2.2.1 Array-CGH

Comparative genomic hybridization (CGH) was developed as a technique for assessing CNA in tumours (Kallioniemi et al., 1992). This technique relies on competitive hybridization of differentially labelled tumour and normal DNA onto a normal metaphase chromosomal preparation. Relative gain and loss are determined by the ratio of fluorophores seen bound to each chromosomal region. In conventional CGH, resolution is limited by the visibility of cytogenetic bands. Array-based CGH is a modification in which the chromosome scaffold is replaced by DNA sequence printed on a microarray. Printed arrays may be comprised of BAC, cDNA, or oligonucleotide probe sequences (Carvalho et al., 2004; Heiskanen et al., 2000; Pinkel et al., 1998; Pollack et al., 1999; Solinas–Toldo et al., 1997). BAC arrays have been designed with tiling genomic coverage based on a set of 32,433 BAC clones spotted in triplicate (Ishkanian et al., 2004). The advantages of full tiling BAC coverage are offset by limitations in specificity of BACs which harbour large spans of repeat sequence or represent regions of genomic duplication. Printed BAC arrays have specific utility in replacing clinical diagnostic based on multi-locus FISH (Bejjani and Shaffer 2006; Cheung et al., 2005; Thorland et al., 2007).

2.2.2 Oligonucleotide arrays

In contrast to printed arrays, more recent technology allows for on-chip synthesis of oligonucleotides at high densities. Non-specific hybridization limits the sensitivity of oligo-aCGH and is a particular concern for methods that directly label total genomic DNA (i.e. full complexity): for every copy of target sequence there are billions of bases on non-target sequence available for partial hybridization. Longer probe sequences have greater specificity and capture more labelled target than short sequences. For direct-labelled genomic DNA (e.g. random prime labelled), oligonucleotides of 50–70 bp are typically used to reduce non-specific hybridization. Several different technologies are currently employed for on-chip synthesis including optical photochemistry (Affymetrix, Nimblegen), 'inkjet' printed chemistry (Agilent) and CMOS on-chip electrochemistry (Combimatrix). Long-oligonucleotide aCGH has been validated for direct genomic labelling and is broadly applied for cancer genomics studies (Barrett et al., 2004; Brennan et al., 2004). On-chip synthesis allows flexibility of probe design, allowing for tiling-resolution of unique genomic sequence or custom design of probesets for specific biologic questions and applications such as chromatin immunoprecipitation, or 'ChIP chip'. Most whole-genome CGH applications utilize pre-printed standardized designs. To support user-specific array design, some manufacturers provide a library of probes which the user can select from. Custom-designed probes are readily printed as well, and careful probe design can improve probe performance (Sharp et al., 2007). Figure 2.1 shows an example of tiling aCGH of a glioblastoma tumour sample using a custom-designed tiling array of 43,000 probes spaced approximately 45 bp apart (excluding genomic repeat sequence). Given the heterogeneity of probe %GC, probe lengths were adjusted between

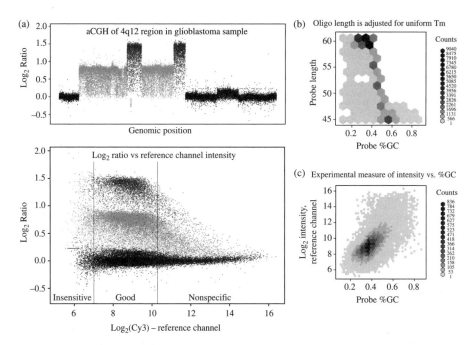

FIG. 2.1: High-density tiling array CGH of a narrow amplicon in a glioblastoma sample (approximately 2 MB region shown). Probes are custom-designed long oligonucleotides (45–60mer) based on unique genome assembly sequence. The amplicon 'signal' allows for analysis of probe performance. (a) Top panel: Probes within regions of apparently uniform copy number are differentially shaped within this complex amplicon. Bottom panel: The same $\log_2$ ratio is plotted as a function of $\log_2$ intensity in the reference channel: Cy3-labelled pooled genomic reference DNA (diploid normal). As expected, probes with the lowest reference channel intensity yield the noisiest estimates of copy number (insensitive hybridization) while the brightest-hybridizing probes show compression of copy number signal (non-specific hybridization). (b) Probe length is trimmed in order to offset variation in %GC of target sequence and thus achieve uniform predicted Tm for the array. (c) Despite Tm correction, probes with the highest %GC content in this design tend to show high-intensity hybridization and performance suggesting non-specific binding. Despite the best informatic design, probe optimization by experimental hybridization is an important step in custom array design.

45–60 bp for uniformity of melting temperature (Fig. 2.1b). $\log_2$ ratios are plotted with differential colouring according to regions of common copy number. Plotting $\log_2$ ratio as a function of reference channel intensity (cy3) reveals the effect of non-specific hybridization in suppressing signal, most prominent in the brighter-hybridizing probes. Despite adjusting probe length to favour uniform melting temperature, a residual effect of %GC on hybridization intensity is seen (Fig. 2.1c). Because probe performance is difficult to predict informatically, a round of experimental optimization is highly valuable – at minimum, discarding highest and lowest intensity probes.

2.2.3 Representational methods

Increasing probe length is one way to ameliorate off-target hybridization. Non-specific hybridization can also be addressed by reducing the complexity of labelled DNA. One approach is to amplify specific target sequences prior to hybridization. Whole Genome Sampling Assay (WGSA) and Representational Oligonucleotide Microarray Analysis (ROMA) are two such approaches which rely on restriction digest followed by linker ligation and PCR of smaller fragments to enrich for defined target sequences (Kennedy et al., 2003; Lucito et al., 2003). In both techniques, the target-enriched amplification product is hybridized to in situ synthesized oligonucleotide arrays. In ROMA, reduced complexity DNA is hybridized to 70mer probes, achieving high specificity of hybridization signal (Lucito et al., 2003).

Reducing complexity allows for use of shorter probe lengths and greater hybridization sensitivity to single-base-pair mismatch. This forms the basis of WGSA as a method for SNP detection as well as copy number estimation as used in the Affymetrix GeneChip platform (Bignell et al., 2004). This single-channel hybridization provides information on total copy number and allelic balance. One disadvantage of this approach is that coverage is dictated by restriction sites. To improve coverage, separate chips may be designed for two or more complementary enzymes. SNP-based profiling has been adapted to bead array technology which favours uniform hybridization in moving liquid environment (Illumina) (Engle et al., 2006). A newer technology, molecular inversion probes or MIP, gains SNP specificity by employing a ligase reaction highly sensitive to SNP mismatch (Wang et al., 2007). MIP arrays are currently being investigated for their performance in calling allele-specific copy number. Representational methods are somewhat limited by noise and artifacts introduced by processes of restriction digest, ligation, and PCR. These artifacts must be carefully monitored and data sets analysed for batch effects. Artifacts from representational arrays may in some cases be reducible by platform-specific algorithmic approaches such as ITALICS and GIM, designed for SNP arrays (Komura et al., 2006; Rigaill et al., 2008).

2.2.4 Digital karyotyping and sequencing-based approaches

Digital karyotyping is a sequencing-based approach to estimate chromosomal copy number (Wang et al., 2002). Short tags (21 bp) are derived using a technique similar to long SAGE, but starting with restriction-fragments of genomic DNA instead of RNA. As in SAGE, tags are concatenated and sequenced. The frequency of 21 bp tag sequences, when mappable to unique genomic sequence, directly represents copy number. This approach can be modified to assess DNA methylation (Hu et al., 2006). As with SAGE, digital karyotyping is limited in sensitivity and resolution by the depth of sequencing, which can be expensive and time-consuming. Massively parallel single-molecule sequencing technologies are increasingly available and competition among platforms is helping reduce costs. These 'next generation' sequencing technologies are just beginning to be applied to the cancer genome (Campbell et al., 2008). It is reasonable to expect that direct sequencing may complement or supplant array-based methods as experience accrues and costs come down. Next-generation platforms currently are most efficient at generating large amounts of short sequences for which assembly (unambiguous mapping) may be greatly aided by an independent measure of copy number. Arrays are likely to remain valuable for high-quality profiling of overall CNA at low cost.

2.3 Choosing a platform: array resolution and practical considerations

As many of the above technologies are rapidly evolving, it is treacherous to generalize about comparative performance and the reader is encouraged to consult the most recent comparison studies (Greshock et al., 2007; Hehir-Kwa et al., 2007). The choice of platform is dictated largely by experimental design and cost considerations. One key decision is whether assaying CNA is the sole objective or if allelic information is important as well. A second decision is what resolution is experimentally required. Because the most prevalent cancer-related CNA is regionally broad gain or loss, the majority of aberration in a tumour sample can be measured by an array with low genomic resolution. Thus measuring global CNA with high probe sensitivity and specificity can be done inexpensively with BAC arrays. Higher genomic resolutions are required to identify narrow CNA events and to resolve their boundaries. Narrow events are rarer but also more informative for identifying cancer-relevant genes targeted by the CNA.

Genomic resolution of a platform is partly defined by probe density and coverage of regions of interest for a particular experiment (e.g. genes vs. intragenic regions). In practice, actual resolution also depends greatly on a number of factors which can be loosely classed as 'signal', 'noise', and 'artifacts'.

A useful definition of 'signal' is the mean copy number (or $\log_2$ ratio) reported by a large population of probes as a function of actual copy number. Factors that affect this measure include average probe sensitivity, specificity and length, DNA amount and labelling efficiency, and the dynamic range of the platform. When the actual copy number (ground truth) is not known, signal may still be compared across platforms. A comparison of signal between long-oligonucleotide array-CGH (Agilent 244K) and short-oligonucleotide SNP/CNA array (Affymetrix 6.0) is shown in Fig. 2.2 and reveals relative compression of $\log_2$ copy number for high-level amplifications in SNP vs. long-oligonucleotide platform. In fact, long oligo arrays also demonstrate signal compression when compared to ground truth copy number determined cytogenetically (Greshock et al., 2007; Hehir-Kwa et al., 2007).

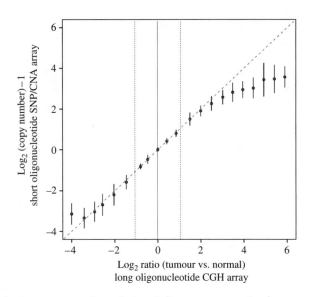

FIG. 2.2: Relative compression of signal ($\log_2$ copy number) compared between two copy number platforms. CNA amplitudes were determined in the same sample set of 84 glioblastoma samples (The Cancer Genome Atlas): 244K long oligonucleotide array (Agilent, $\log_2$ ratio, tumour vs. normal) and short oligonucleotide SNP/CNA array (Affymetrix SNP 6.0, $\log_2$ copy number/2). Relative compression in the short oligo platform is evident for larger amplitude amplifications and deletions (outside dotted lines). Signal compression is present in all microarray-based approaches. Ideally, platform performance should be compared to cytogenetically defined standards of absolute copy number.

If 'signal' is defined as the mean of individual probe copy number estimates across a uniform region, a practical definition of 'noise' should capture the variance of these individual probe values across regions of uniform copy number. Factors affecting 'noise' include DNA amplification or representation steps, imperfections in the array, hybridization uniformity, array imaging, and also the variation in performance between individual probes. Platform noise can be estimated by the standard deviation of probe values after subtracting the regional mean, defined either by a moving window or by segmentation procedure. Alternatively, noise can be simply estimated by standard deviation of the differences between $\log_2$ ratios of neighbouring probes (scaled by square root of 2), since most neighbouring probes measure identical underlying copy number.

Studies that directly compare platform performance may use a common set of cell lines and regions of well-defined copy number (based on cytogenetics) to establish the ground-truth CNA being measured. Probe performance can be characterized by a signal-to-noise model or by analyses of detection power such as receiver operating characteristic (ROC) curves (Greshock et al., 2007; Hehir-Kwa et al., 2007).

Noise can be greatly reduced by averaging copy number estimates from neighbouring probes within a region of uniform CNA. Therefore a natural definition of practical array resolution can be phrased as the number of probes which must be averaged together to achieve a fixed sensitivity and specificity for detection of a fixed copy number change (such as single copy loss or gain), times the median genomic interval between probes. An example of such an analysis is shown in Fig. 2.3. In this example, a single tumour sample is hybridized against two long oligo CGH arrays with 42,500 and 231,000 mapped features, designated '44K' and '244K' arrays, respectively. ROC curves are plotted for detection of two-fold copy number change between chr1 and chrX. A specificity of 99% is chosen arbitrarily, understanding that higher specificity would be needed for single probe calls on a large array to avoid excessive false positives. ROC curves are plotted for raw $\log_2$ ratios as well as increasing numbers of averaged probes. The per-probe sensitivity for this test is 64% for the 44K array and 93% for the 244K. To achieve a sensitivity of >98%, four probes must be averaged from the 44K array versus two probes for the 244K platform. Giving median interprobe intervals of 37.6kb and 9.7kb, respectively, the 44K and 244K arrays have a practical resolution of approximately 150kb and 19kb for two-fold gain. Actual comparison of platform resolution must be made with multiple samples, preferably with replicates. Such performance-based measures are an important factor in choosing between platforms, though it should also be recognized that platform performance can vary greatly between different samples, core facilities, and even days the hybridizations are performed.

2.4 Segmentation

Fundamental to the analysis of copy number data is the underlying model of chromosomal aberration: that copy number is uniform over a genomic region and then jumps abruptly at transition points. A set of probes hybridizing to genomic targets within a span of uniform copy number is essentially redundant and their individual estimates can be combined to reduce noise. Segmentation or changepoint algorithms apply such models to the raw data in order to localize and quantify CNAs and their transition boundaries. Segmentation allows greater resolution of CNA events that span several probes and reduces false positives, albeit at the cost of false negative calls for extremely narrow events. A diversity of algorithms has been developed and applied to copy number data. The moving average or median filter is a simple approach to combining individual probe estimates and can be coupled to thresholding to determine boundaries of CNA, albeit inexactly. Circular Binary Segmentation (CBS) is a changepoint detection technique which attempts to find boundaries around a uniform distribution of probe values by maximum likelihood and permutation-based significance testing (R package 'DNAcopy') (Olshen et al., 2004; Venkatraman and Olshen, 2007).

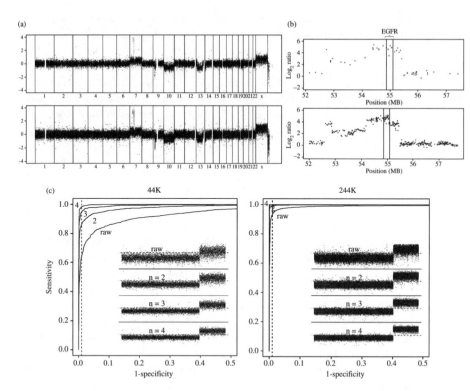

FIG. 2.3: Receiver Operating Characteristic (ROC) analysis with n-neighbour averaging of probe $\log_2$ ratios: a systematic approach to defining and comparing useful platform resolution. (a) Example comparative profiles of same tumour DNA sample on two long oligonucleotide array-CGH platforms of differing resolution: ~44K probes (top) vs. ~244K (bottom). (b) Zoom-in of chromosome 7, 52–57MB. Increased coverage is apparent when the profile is inspected closely. EGFR gene boundaries marked by vertical lines. (c) ROC analysis for 44K and 244K platforms detecting single-copy loss vs. euploidy, for various windows of n-neighbour probe averaging. Insert figures show data sampled from the profiles in (a), from regions of single copy loss and diploidy, after averaging n-nearest neighbouring probes. Reduction in noise with averaging approximates the square root law. Threshold is shown for 99% detection specificity (dashed lines). For 44K data, raw $\log_2$ ratios show only ~60% sensitivity for detecting single copy loss. Sensitivity is increased to 98% if four probes are averaged, though at the direct cost of genomic resolution. In this example, the 244K array has better baseline performance with raw $\log_2$ ratios showing ~93% sensitivity at 99% specificity. Averaging two neighbouring probes suffices to achieve >98% sensitivity. Note that for an array with 250,000 spots, a specificity as high as 99% still predicts 2500 false positive events reported.

Examples of other approaches (many available as downloadable packages) are those based on hidden Markov models (Marioni et al., 2006; Stjernqvist et al., 2007), clustering (Wang et al., 2005; Xing et al., 2007), adaptive weights smoothing (Hupe et al., 2004), and Wavelet fitting (Hsu et al., 2005). Evaluating the performance of these algorithms is problematic since differences in platform noise and resolution, sample type and labelling artifacts can vary considerably. Extensive cross-platform comparisons are lacking and more importantly, 'ground truth' of chromosomal aberrations is typically unknown even for exemplary samples, particularly at finer scales. Lai and colleagues have directly compared the performance of eleven different algorithms for localizing CNA using aCGH data (Lai et al., 2005). In this comparison, the segmentation-based methods CBS and CGHseg (Picard et al., 2005) performed well throughout a range of signal-to-noise. This same group has made their comparative analysis available as a web-based tool, CGHweb, which allows users to upload their own data to directly compare the results of a panel of segmentation algorithms (Lai et al., 2008).

If it seems that there is an excess of methods for segmenting CGH data, it is worth remembering that their performance differs most in the detection of narrow events and their sensitivity to noise and artifacts in the data. One algorithm may call an event real that another rejects as spurious. Because researchers may be quick to invest time and resources pursuing functional studies for genes that appear to be targeted by narrow events, it is imperative to understand the performance of segmentation approaches in this domain. For all segmentation approaches it can be particularly useful to have an idea of the confidence with which a CNA has been detected and also an error range or distribution associated with localizing each boundary. Some algorithms, such as CBS, include these confidence and error scores, which are useful for prioritizing loci and resolving discrepancies between experiments and across platforms.

2.4.1 Artifacts

Noise that varies independently across probes can be addressed by averaging and by the automated segmentation methods described in the next section. However, when a source of noise affects two or more adjacent probes coordinately it is often not possible to distinguish from real CNA. The presence of genomic regional artifacts in a copy number profile is therefore a particularly insidious problem, and the nature of artifacts for any platform should be well-understood before profiles are analysed for copy number aberration. There are several possible sources of artifact. Uneven genomic fragmentation, fragment labelling, genome amplification, or PCR can introduce fluctuations in the profile which are regionally correlated and which may suggest actual CNA. An example of a genomic regional artifact is shown in Fig. 2.4. The profile shows waves embedded in the $\log_2$ ratio which are mistakenly identified as regional CNA by segmentation. This artifact is correlated with mean %GC calculated by a 20KB moving window across the genome. The artifact is also correlated with 2KB and 50KB window moving averages. This form of artifact has been seen in copy number data sets from both

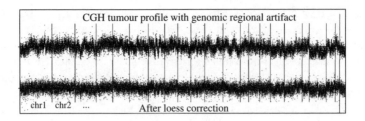

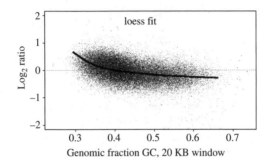

FIG. 2.4: Genomic regional artifacts are can potentially be mistaken for real CNA. An example of an aCGH profile which is nearly entirely artifactual is shown (top). The 'waves' in $\log_2$ ratio are suggestive of complex CNA but are in fact highly correlated with genomic %GC averaged in windows of 2–50KB around probe locations. These artifacts can arise from a variety of sources, and can be detected by correlation with genomic %GC models during data QC. Multidimensional loess, described in the text, can significantly reduce this form of artifact.

aCGH and SNP-based platforms. In practice, we measure the artifact amplitude (covariance with %GC models) as part of QC and apply multidimensional loess to reduce the amplitude in the raw $\log_2$ ratios before segmentation.

2.5 Aberration types

2.5.1 *Regional and focal aberrations*

While there is no standard nomenclature for CNA in the literature, there is a common convention of naming CNA by degree which is followed in this chapter: 'homozygous deletion' or simply 'deletion' refers to complete deletion of a chromosomal region; 'heterozygous deletion' or 'loss' refers to loss of one copy out of two; 'gain' typically refers to the addition of one or two extra copies; and 'amplification' is reserved for copy numbers >4. The distinction between low-level gain/loss and higher-impact amplification/deletion extends beyond the number of copies counted and reflects an important aspect of CNA in cancer: gain and loss are common and most often involve extended regions (>10MB) whereas amplifications and homozygous deletions are typically rarer and more focal.

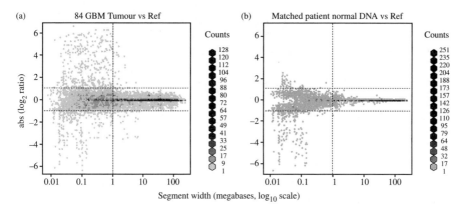

FIG. 2.5: Typical relationship of CNA amplitude to CNA width in an aCGH profiling data set. DNA from 84 glioblastoma tumours and matching normal DNA from blood were hybridized separately against a pooled genomic DNA reference. Raw $\log_2$ ratios were processed by Circular Binary Segmentation. (a) 2-D histogram of the absolute values of mean $\log_2$ ratios after segmentation, plotted as a function of segment width, in 84 GBM tumour profiles. Most segments are long and near zero $\log_2$ ratio (euploid). Low amplitude gain/loss events ($|\log_2 \text{ratio}| < 1$, horizontal dashed lines) account for a majority of CNA and are typically broad (>1MB, vertical line). High amplitude amplifications and deletions ($|\log_2 \text{ratio}| > 1$) tend to be focal (<1MB). (b) Matching normal DNA (blood) from the same patients shows a substantial number of narrow segments with non-diploid copy number. Some of these events appear to be artifactual, a result of trends in $\log_2$ ratio aberrantly identified as CNA (see Fig. 4). The majority, however, map either to known regions of copy number variation in the general population or to genomic regions variably deleted during immune globulin and receptor rearrangement in leukocytes. The latter are exposed when hybridizing blood-derived DNA to pooled genomic reference DNA derived from non-blood tissues or placenta.

Figure 2.5 shows a typical distribution of CNA widths and amplitudes for a set of 84 glioblastoma tumour samples and their matched normals, each hybridized against a common pooled genomic DNA reference (The Cancer Genome Atlas Research Network, 2008). The $\log_2$ ratio copy number profiles have been processed by Circular Binary Segmentation to identify spans of uniform copy number. Regional gain and loss ($|\log_2 \text{ratio}|$ between ~0.2 and 1.0) are prevalent and include many long segments, mean width 8MB. Among tumours, 7.5% of the CNA events are amplifications and deletions ($|\log_2 \text{ratio}| > 1.0$) and nearly all are narrow (<1MB). These focal events span an average of 400KB and include 3–4 genes on average. In this example, 660 genes and miRNAs are within such amplified or deleted regions. Some of these genes are focally targeted in multiple tumours: 144 genes are altered in more than 5% of the tumours and the top gene, amplified in 58% of GBM samples, is the tyrosine kinase receptor EGFR. The most recurrent deleted gene is the Ink4a/ARF locus (38%). Figure 2.5(b) shows the same analysis run on the 84 matching normal DNA samples against the same reference DNA. Note that many narrow events are found in the blood-derived DNA and these are mostly accounted for by a combination of copy number polymorphisms in the general population as well as genomic regions commonly deleted in leukocyte pools, such and immunoglobulin and immune receptor subunits.

2.5.2 Copy number variation

Analysis of the human genome has revealed a surprising degree of copy number variation between individuals (CNV) (Sebat et al., 2004; Redon et al., 2006; Freeman et al., 2006). CNV regions represent spans of the genome sequence that are variably present or variably duplicated in the genome among individuals. It has been estimated that as much as 12% of the human genome is present in variable copy number (Carter 2007). Compared to SNP, CNV prevalence in the general population is poorly characterized. Comparative analysis of genome assemblies or sequence shows CNV may be associated with genomic rearrangements and represent one of a diversity of classes and scales of variation in the genome (Khaja et al., 2006; Sharp et al., 2005). Based on sequence homology, a CNV region may not have discrete, well-defined endpoints in the genome. Current studies of population CNV report the location of probes or markers which were differential in copy number between individuals, and the reported 'boundaries' of the CNV are inferred inexactly from probe/marker positions. Therefore CNV databases that compile reported events are currently incomplete and with inexact boundaries; they should be used with caution. With those caveats noted, compiled databases of reported CNV, such as the Database of Genomic Variants (http://projects.tcag.ca/variation/), can be a useful reference for approximate positions of common polymorphisms found in the general population so far (Iafrate et al., 2004).

Fine-mapping of CNV breakpoints can be accomplished by sequencing and it is expected that a more complete database of variation in the human genome will follow the growth of large-scale genomic sequencing projects with 'next generation' sequencing technologies (Korbel et al., 2007).

An understanding of CNV is critical to interpreting copy number data in cancer profiling. Because they are both recurrent across samples and focal, unrecognized germline CNV may masquerade as attractive copy number aberrations. Ideally, experimental design will include correction for germline CNV by profiling patient-matched germline DNA separately or as a reference in two-colour hybridizations. As demonstrated in Fig. 2.1, it should be noted that DNA derived from blood inexactly matches germline DNA due to heterogeneous functional deletions in immune receptor and immunoglobulin loci among leukocytes. In experiments where matched normal is not available, one can expect a significant number of CNVs to be evident in the copy number profile. CNAs that match known locations of copy number polymorphism in the general population are likely to be germline events. However, the possibility of somatically acquired aberration in a region of known CNV must be considered. A recent report of differential copy number between identical twins supports the view that rearrangements leading to CNV are perhaps common (Bruder et al., 2008). Finally, CNVs are associated with altered expression and CNVs found overrepresented in a cancer data set may include susceptibility loci (Stranger et al., 2007).

2.5.3 Regional/broad CNA

As exemplified in Fig. 2.5, broad regions of gain and loss are the most common form of CNA found in cancer profiling data sets. Gain and loss often involve entire chromosomes or chromosomal arms. The pattern of gain and loss is typically tumour-type specific, forming patterns familiar to the cytogeneticist. The tumour-specific pattern may represent clonal selection of an advantageous gene dosage alteration generated by background genomic instability and spread over thousands of genes. The gain/loss patterns may also indicate molecularly defined tumour subclasses (Carrasco et al., 2006; Maher et al., 2006). The broadly distributed nature of gain and loss often frustrates efforts to determine the underlying biological cause. For example, glioblastoma shows a high incidence of gain of the whole of chromosome 7. Presumably tumour cells with this pattern have a growth advantage conferred by increased dosage of at least one gene, but hundreds of genes on the chromosome may be equally implicated. Integration of other data sets such as expression profiling, epigenetic, mutation, or functional genomic assays can be useful to further narrow the list of candidate targets (Tonon et al., 2005). Through such an integrated analysis, one study has found evidence that chromosome 7 gain in glioblastoma may in some cases be driven by the effects of simultaneous gain of the MET tyrosine kinase receptor and its ligand, HGF, which both reside on 7 (Beroukhim et al., 2007).

2.5.4 Focal CNA

It is perhaps obvious that copy number aberrations which are focal are the most tractable for identifying the candidate genes, miRNAs or other genetic elements being targeted. Current microarray technologies based on hundreds of thousands of probes can readily detect CNA spanning a single gene or even a region internal to the gene. A properly vetted list of focal CNAs culled from cancer genome profiling can directly drive validation experiments, and there are numerous examples of oncogenes and tumour suppressors being identified from this starting point. However, the researcher is advised to move cautiously. First, a single CNA event can often show complex composition which defies simple estimation of the width of the event and the portion of the genome targeted. Figure 2.6 highlights a diversity of CNA morphologies which must be considered. Four aCGH profiles of glioblastoma are shown from the TCGA data set (The Cancer Genome Atlas Network, 2008), with a second panel highlighting region 12q14-15. The first profile has a split chr12 amplicon spanning 67.0–67.6MB

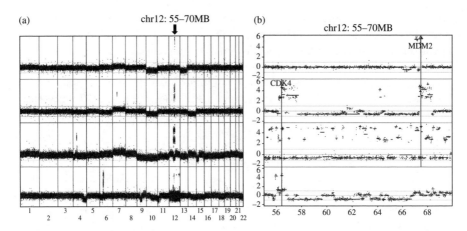

FIG. 2.6: Array-CGH of four glioblastoma tumours selected to demonstrate increasing complexity of CNA on chromosome 12. Raw $\log_2$ ratios (black dots) and segmentation results (black lines) are shown for the whole genome (a) and for a chr12 region harbouring several proto-oncogenes including CDK4 and MDM2 (b, gene positions marked). In the first profile, a single narrow complex amplicon targets four genes, including MDM2. Subsequent profiles demonstrate greater disruption and complexity with additional plausible targets such as CDK4. These complex amplicons are likely physically joined in double-minute chromosome fragments though they appear discontiguous when plotted by genomic position. Analytical approaches to summarizing CNA across samples must contend with a wide range of CNA topographies and correlations of CNA events which may map to discontiguous genomic regions.

with internal deletion 67.2–67.47MB. Such narrow split amplicons are likely to be physically joined (in this case in a double-minute chromosome fragment) with the internal deletion as a result of recombination. This paired amplicon spans four genes including MDM2, a direct inactivator of p53 and plausible target of the amplicon. The second profile shows a more complex picture with two main amplicons, each showing multiple internal copy number transitions. Again, it is likely that these amplicons both reside on a common chromosomal fragment. Should these be considered a single linked event targeting all genes spanned by the pair, two independent complex events, or multiple independent events of differing amplitudes? The third and fourth profiles show further degrees of complexity, with the latter showing extensive rearrangement of the entire chromosome.

Even for simple topographies, focal CNA candidates must be carefully vetted before inferring biological significance. As described above, focal CNA is readily mimicked by germline copy number variation. Experiments should include analysis of matched normal DNA and lists of focal CNA should be compared to databases of known CNV. CNA may also be mimicked by systematic array artifacts and genomic labelling artifacts described previously. Finally, as with point mutations, some focal CNA may point to cancer-relevant genes while others are random 'passenger' events: aberrations which are clonally propagated but do not themselves confer a growth advantage.

2.6 Assigning significance to CNA

Gene resequencing studies in cancer have led to the development of statistical methods for determining 'driver' SNP mutations from a background of 'passenger' events (Greenman et al., 2007; Wood et al., 2007). These methods rely on a background model for passenger point mutation, derived in part from the prevalence of silent or synonymous SNPs of various forms. Can a similar approach be used to define driver CNA mutations? This is complicated for at least three reasons: (1) there is no realistic model for the background process of CNA in cancer; (2) unlike SNP mutation, CNA covers many genes, is highly spatially correlated, often with complex topography; and (3) there is no CNA equivalent to synonymous events; no systematic methods to assign potential biological significance to CNA. Several approaches have been proposed, largely based on measuring amplitude, focality and recurrence of CNAs overlapping across samples, testing against a null model to attempt to distinguish driver events. The methods differ primarily in what assumptions are made in defining CNAs, determining overlap across data sets and modelling the background CNA rate typically by non-parametric methods. As highlighted in Fig. 2.6, the topography of CNA presents a vastly more complex problem determining driver CNA events compared to point mutations. Three approaches will be described here.

'Significance Testing for Aberrant Copy-Number' (STAC) analyses regions of aberration defined by reducing continuous copy number data to discrete calls of 'aberrant' and 'normal' (done for gains and losses separately) (Diskin et al., 2006). 'Stacks' of aberrations that overlap recurrently across samples are then analysed to generate two statistics for each point in the genome: frequency-based and footprint-based. A frequency score is computed for each genomic region essentially as the count of samples which have aberration at each point. This score is tested for significance based on positional permutation of aberration regions in the data, yielding a frequency-based p-value, P_{fr}. The frequency score does not consider the width of the aberrations and so does not distinguish focal from broad events. A complementary 'footprint' p-value is designed to address this by considering the width (footprint) of sets of aberrations that are overlapping across samples and computing a likelihood based on a null model. The computation is complicated by the need to consider all combinations of overlapping aberrations which span a genomic position. If five samples have aberrations spanning a particular position, footprint scores must be considered for the complete set as well as each possible combination of two, three, and four samples. The result is a p-value for the best footprint seen (narrowest overlap among largest subset of samples). An optimization strategy is employed to tame the computation which is otherwise exponential with sample size. The two p-values, P_{fr} and

P_{fp}, can be used to survey the genome for loci of recurrent and focal aberrations. The amplitude of CNA is not considered by the original STAC approach, other than by initial thresholds used to define 'aberration'. The authors have extended their approach to consider a range of thresholds, including appropriate correction for multiple testing (Guttman et al., 2007). This Multiple Sample Analysis (MSA) algorithm allows for automatic selection of thresholds which best capture signal-to-noise in each genomic region separately – reflecting an important aspect of CNA which is often distributed unevenly across chromosomal regions. MSA has significantly increased computational time compared to STAC. The authors determine performance using a simulated data model that is also publically available. One limitation of STAC/MSA is that all non-contiguous CNA regions within a profile are treated as independent events, whereas physical linkage of genomically discontinuous CNA, as seen in Fig. 2.6, is common.

A second approach, Genomic Identification of Significant Targets in Cancer (GISTIC), analyses a set of copy number profiles to compute a score ('G score') for each genomic region: essentially the sum of the $\log_2$ ratios for samples which show aberration, considering gains and losses separately (Beroukhim et al., 2007). The G scores are compared to the distribution seen with positional permutation (within chromosome or chromosomal arm) and significantly altered regions are identified. GISTIC then applies some additional heuristics aimed at better-resolving regions that are independently targeted by CNA. First, significant regions are recalculated with a leave-one-out strategy to generate conservative boundaries. For each chromosomal arm, the most significantly altered (peak) region is noted. G scores are then recalculated after leaving out all samples that showed CNA in the peak region, and the next peak region is identified. This 'peel off' strategy is repeated until no significant peaks remain. Unlike STAC, GISTIC does not model CNA focality explicitly, though 'focal' vs. 'broad' events are distinguished based on their width relative to the chromosomal arm length and are analysed in separate runs.

The p- and q-values returned by STAC and GISTIC are based on models of background CNA derived from permutation and sampling of the cancer profile data set. The resulting statistics are generally quite conservative, and potentially informative CNAs are missed if they fall below the significance thresholds for recurrence. For example, in a set of 205 glioblastoma tumour profiles from the TCGA, the p53 tumour suppressor is found focally deleted in only one sample. While the single event is not statistically significant alone, integration of additional data (namely LOH and expression) readily identifies p53 as a candidate target of frequent silencing in GBM. In order to identify such informative rare events we have developed an approach, Genome Topography Survey (GTS), which scores three essential features of CNA across a data set of CNA profiles: frequency, amplitude, and focality (Wiedemeyer et al., 2008). GTS assigns two scores for each genomic position: Aberration Recurrence Index (ARI) and Aberration Focality Index (AFI). ARI is essentially identical to the GISTIC G score above, and captures the frequency and amplitude of CNA across samples.

ARI for gain events is calculated as the sum of the $\log_2$ ratios of all samples gained at the genomic position (a separate score is calculated for loss events). Amplitude and recurrence are combined: high score at a particular position may arise from summing many samples with moderate CNA amplitude at that location or few samples with high amplitude CNA. Note that as with GISTIC's G score and STAC's P_{fr}, high ARI values provide no information about how often CNA was seen focally targeting the region. For this reason, the complementary Aberration Focality Index (AFI) is derived by considering the widths of the overlapping CNA events, and applying a model for linkage which accounts for complex CNAs such as shown in Fig. 2.6. AFI represents what proportion of the ARI score is distributed across potential target genes or other genetic elements in the region. As with ARI, AFI is calculated for each genomic position, separately for gained and lost sample subsets. Focality is determined by one of three models for potential linkage of CNA across the profile: *local linkage* treats each group of adjacent gained (or lost) segments as part of a discrete amplicon (or deletion) implying a set of target genetic elements spanned by the adjacent segments; *chromosome linkage* considers that non-adjacent CNAs within the same chromosome represent a single amplicon (or deletion) with a shared set of targets; *genome linkage* treats all CNA as if it potentially belongs to a single complex rearrangement. Genome linkage is the most conservative model, though not likely to be biologically accurate in most cases. Local linkage may overreport focality for complex CNA. Chromosomal linkage is a compromise which appears to best capture the kind of intrachromosomal rearrangement shown in Fig. 2.6. The method for calculating focality is shown schematically in Fig. 2.7 and is described as follows:

For each segment $S_{i=1..N_{\text{total}}}$ in a CNA profile of N_{total} segments:

S_i^{mean} = mean $\log_2$ ratio for segment i

S_i^{elements} = number of genomic elements spanned by segment genomic start/end (or 1 if no elements are spanned).

Groups of linked segments, S_{G_1}, S_{G_2}, etc., are determined by the linkage model:

Genome linkage: one group, S_G, comprised of all gained (or lost) segments;

Chromosome linkage: 24 groups, $S_{G_{1..24}}$, of all gained (or lost) segments per chromosome;

Local linkage: M groups, $S_{G_{1..M}}$, of contiguous gained (or lost) segments bounded by non-gained segments or chromosomal ends.

Then for each group of segments, S_{G_n}, the N segments are ordered ($1 < i < N$) by increasing $|S_i^{\text{mean}}|$. The segment focality-weighted mean, fwMean, is then

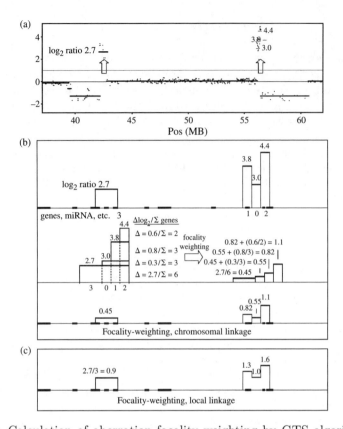

FIG. 2.7: Calculation of aberration focality weighting by GTS algorithm. The goal is to reweight CNA events by their width, measured by the number of genetic elements (genes, miRNAs, etc.) or base pairs spanned by the event. (a) Example glioblastoma CNA profile from chr12 is shown with $\log_2$ ratio (grey points) and segmentation (black lines). Two amplicons are seen (open arrows), each associated with neighbouring regions of loss. The amplicon at 56MB is complex, with three segmented subregions. (b) Schematic of the same aCHG profile showing calculation of focality-weighted segment means by the chromosomal linkage model. In this conservative model, genomically discontiguous events on the same chromosome are considered part of the same physical CNA. For each amplified segment, the mean $\log_2$ ratio is determined as well as the count of genes spanned (grey lines, numbers). The segments are then joined and ordered by ascending amplitude. For each rising plateau of $\log_2$ ratio, the step increase is divided by the total genes spanned at-or-above that level. The segments are assigned weights based on the cumulative sum of the ratios. Aberration Focality Index (AFI) is then computed by summing these reweighted segment values at each genomic position across a set of the sample (further described in the text). Focality weighting can be based on the number of genetic elements spanned by CNA, as in this example, or by the genomic length in base-pairs. (c) Calculation by local linkage model considers the two amplicons to be independently targeting two separate regions. Compared to chromosomal linkage in (b), both amplicons are assigned higher focality weights.

calculated for each segment in the group by:

$$S_i^{\text{fwMean}} = \frac{\left(S_i^{\text{mean}} - S_{i-1}^{\text{mean}}\right)}{\sum_{j=i}^{N} S_j^{\text{elements}}} + \sum_{k=1}^{i-1} S_k^{\text{fwMean}}.$$

After all profiles have been analysed, focality-weighted ARI (fwARI) is calculated as for ARI, but using the S^{fwMean} of each segment instead of mean log$_2$ ratio, S^{mean}. Then AFI = fwARI/ARI.

The two scores, ARI and AFI, can be combined to rank genomic regions by the degree to which they are targeted by focal, recurrent, and high-amplitude CNAs. These scores can also be compared to the distribution of scores obtained after positional permutation of the data set. However, the primary goal of GTS is to identify discrete genomic regions worthy of further investigation, either by integration of additional genomic, bioinformatic, or functional data. Results for GTS analysis of glioma copy number profiling are shown in Fig. 2.8. Validation is suggested by the high GTS ranking of both known glioma-relevant cancer genes and several tumour suppressors not previously implicated in glioma, and since functionally validated: p18/CDKN2C, PTPRD and NF1 (Wiedemeyer et al., 2008; Solomon et al., 2008; The Cancer Genome Atlas Network, 2008).

GTS scoring is reproducible across copy number microarray platforms. In the preliminary analysis of the TCGA data set for glioblastoma, genes and miRNAs were ranked by GTS scores derived from a common set of 139 tumours analysed by array-CGH (Agilent 244K Whole Genome CGH Array) and SNP platforms (Affymetrix SNP 6.0). Regions of known or suspected copy number variation

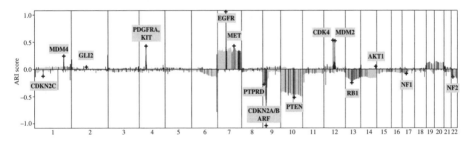

FIG. 2.8: GTS multi-sample analysis of glioblastoma aCGH profiles reveals focal and recurrent CNA targeting oncogenes and tumour suppressors known to be implicated in GBM, as well as new genes not previously identified as targets of deletion in GBM such as tumour suppressors CDKN2C, NF1 and PTPRD. GTS ARI score is shown plotted in grey, calculated separately for gains and losses (assigned positive an negative sign, respectively). Black slices mark regions of highest AFI score (top 5%ile). Peaks in ARI which are also focally targeted (high AFI) are enriched for cancer-relevant genes. GTS is one strategy for multi-sample copy number analysis described in the text.

(CNV) were excluded. The 200 genes with top-ranked GTS scores in the aCGH data set were compared to the GTS rankings derived from the SNP data set. For amplifications, 78% of the top 200 aCGH-identified genes were ranked within the top 400 SNP-identified genes. For deletions, the comparable overlap was 63%. Among the top 200 altered genes are nearly all oncogenes and tumour suppressors known to be implicated in glioma. Overall enrichment for cancer-relevant genes was assessed by Fisher's exact test, considering the subset of genes from the Cancer Gene Census which did not reside in regions of known or suspected CNV. There was significant overrepresentation of cancer relevant genes in these focally altered gene sets, as assessed by comparison with the Cancer Gene Census list (Futreal et al., 2004), both for amplified (odds ratio 7.34, $p < 0.00001$) and deleted genes (odds ratio 3.5, $p = 0.01$).

2.7 Breakpoints/translocations

For genomic DNA in the cell nucleus, naked double-strand breaks are unstable and subject to non-homologous end joining (NHEJ) (Ferguson et al., 2000). Transitions in copy number (say from a region of two copies to three copies) imply either a double-strand break with NHEJ or a homology-based recombination. That is, virtually all copy number transitions (CNT) are associated with novel DNA junctions. The converse is true only for unbalanced events. Most junctions will be between non-coding regions or will produce an out-of-frame coding sequence that will not yield a functional fusion transcript. However, in some cases CNT may mark unbalanced translocations associated with promoter swap or functional gene fusion as seen with TMPRSS-ERG (Hermans et al., 2006; Liu et al., 2007). Gene fusions may also be associated with intrachromosomal deletions, such as seen with FIP1L1-PDGFRA fusion in hypereosinophilic syndrome (Cools et al., 2003). Copy-number data can be used to assay for unbalanced rearrangements associated with gene fusion and translocation in this fashion. Figure 2.9(a) demonstrates aCGH detection of single-copy and homozygous 5' gene end deletions associated with known TK gene fusions FIP1L1-PDGFRA and FIG-ROS1, respectively. Using this approach, we have identified several novel TK gene fusions in glioblastoma including a dual fusion of two TK genes: KDR and PDGFRA (Fig. 2.9(b)). The copy number profile is inspected to identify transitions taking place within genes. While some of these events are associated with fusions, most represent chance events. This is understood by considering that approximately 25% of the genome is exonic or intronic and therefore the chance of a random CNT being intragenic is equally high. In order to distinguish events occurring more frequently than by chance, a statistical model can be employed based on the gene size and background distribution of CNTs. We have developed an R package to perform this ranking of intragenic CNT in segmented copy number data (iCNA, http://cbio.mskcc.org/brennan). Access to exon-level expression data on the same samples can help discriminate intragenic CNA events that lead to actual altered transcripts. An example of this coordinate analysis is shown in Fig. 2.10.

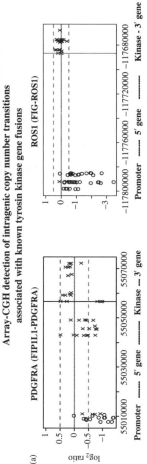
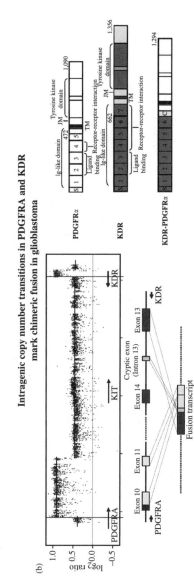

FIG. 2.9: Detection of unbalanced chromosomal events associated with gene fusion and/or translocation by array-CGH. (a) Proof of principal detection of gene fusions of PDGFRA and ROS1 known to be associated with 5′ gene end deletions of one copy and both copies, respectively. 75 long oligonucleotide aCGH probes are designed for the promoter, 5′ coding and 3′ coding regions of each gene. Probes show variable performance but clearly detect the deletions preserving the kinase domain (grey vertical line). (b) Fine mapping of breakpoints by high-density tiling array-CGH (above) identifies intragenic copy number transitions in both PDGFRA and KDR in a glioblastoma sample. Fine mapping enables design of PCR primers spanning putative KDR-PDGFRA fusion site. Sequencing confirms chimeric fusion by rearrangement including cryptic exon from KDR intron 13. The fusion is within the Ig-like domains of both RTKs (upper right). The junction demonstrates eight base pairs of identical sequence between KDR cryptic exon and PDGFRA exon 10.

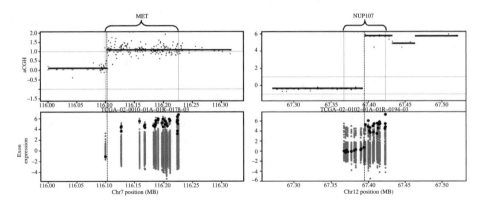

FIG. 2.10: Integration of high-resolution copy number profiling and exon expression enables detection of intragenic rearrangements which lead to altered transcripts. Amplification of the MET tyrosine appears to exclude the native promoter and first exon. Elevated exon expression is noted for this sample (black dots) versus other GBM samples (grey), except for the first exon which shows low expression. Similarly, differential expression of 5' and 3' exons is seen in NUP107 which aligns with an intragenic copy number transition.

2.8 Clustering approaches

Copy number data can be analysed with supervised and unsupervised clustering methods. However, copy number data has essential differences when compared with expression data and these must be taken into account when planning and interpreting cluster analysis.

One fundamental difference is that most copy number alteration is low-level gain and loss, and the gene copy 'signal' driving clustering is of low amplitude compared to gene expression data, in which transcript copies can vary over several orders of magnitude. Artifacts such as those related to genomic labelling, uneven WGA or PCR, can comprise a significant portion of the overall variance of a copy number profile and may dominate clustering, particularly for correlation-based metrics. Euclidean or other distance metrics may be less susceptible. Principal component analysis (PCA) may be useful to isolate artifactual components and remove them from the data. Segmentation is often critical to perform prior to clustering to reduce artifacts. A second fundamental difference between CNA and expression data is that virtually all CNA events are regional – most probes are redundantly measuring the same copy number in each sample as their neighbouring probes in the genome. Thus there are multiple reasonable approaches to assigning weights to features in clustering – one is not restricted to clustering a full length vector representing CNA estimates at the platform probe locations. A third difference lies in the interpretation of the data: genomic gains and losses are biologically distinct events, not simply 'more or less' gene copies. In fact, it is not clear if a 10-copy focal amplicon seen in one sample is biologically different from a 50-copy amplicon of the same region in another sample: both are evidence of selective targeting of the genes spanned, and both are thought to be biologically significant compared to the euploid two-copy state.

We have developed an approach to clustering with non-negative matrix factorization which attempts to address these differences (Carrasco et al., 2006; Maher et al., 2006). The data are first made non-negative by replacing each probe $\log_2$ ratio estimate V_n with a pair of variables (V_n^g, V_n^l) where $V_n^g = \max(0, V_n)$ and $V_n^l = \max(0, -V_n)$. This effectively doubles the length of the profile and separates loss events from gain events as distinct non-exclusive features for clustering. To address the redundancy of most probes, the data may optionally be dimension-reduced by selecting the subset of genomic locations with uniform copy number across all samples. Clustering is performed by non-negative matrix factorization (Brunet et al., 2004). Like PCA, NMF is a matrix decomposition which is designed to return components which account for decreasing variance in the data. However, NMF components are constrained by requiring only positive features (non-negative) rather than the constraint of orthogonality in PCA. It is reasonable to interpret CNA events, whether deletions or amplifications, as distinct positive features. Compared to K-means, PCA and hierarchical clustering, we have found NMF to return components and cluster assignments which are more readily interpretable and better correlate with clinical and pathological parameters. Figure 2.11 shows the results of NMF in a data set of multiple

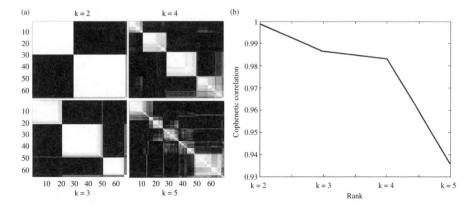

FIG. 2.11: Genomic non-negative matrix factorization (gNMF) applied to a multiple myeloma aCGH dataset (Carrasco et al., 2006). gNMF is a method of data reduction and unsupervised clustering designed for copy number data (Brunet et al., 2004; Maher et al., 2006). Shown are consensus matrices for 1000 iterations of gNMF: grayscale denotes percent of iterations in which samples pairs were assigned to the same clusters: white marks sample pairs always assigned to the same classes while black marks sample pairs always assigned to different classes. In this study, a two-, three- and four-way classifications are stable and fit the data well, measured by cophenetic correlation.

myeloma, finding evidence for division of tumours into three-way and four-way subclasses. These subclasses, defined by NMF components harbouring specific features in the copy number profile, were found to have prognostic significance (Carrasco et al., 2006).

2.9 Conclusion

Technologies for assessing chromosomal copy number continue to rapidly evolve, as do the methods for analysing this form of genomic profiling data. Many of the complexities in analysis transcend platform considerations and are likely to be relevant even if copy number is ultimately assessed by direct sequencing of cancer genomes. Understanding copy number variation and artifacts is critical to interpreting cancer genome profiling. Gene rearrangements such as translocations, fusions, and intragenic deletions are increasingly evident as resolutions improve. Systematic approaches to identifying CNA recurrence across a sample set, whether focused on broad events, focal events or intragenic aberrations, can greatly simplify a complex cancer genome, yielding a prioritized set of regions for further investigation.

References

Barrett, M. T., et al. (2004), Comparative genomic hybridization using oligonucleotide microarrays and total genomic DNA, *Proc. Natl. Acad. Sci. USA*, **101**(51), 17765–70.

Bejjani, B. A. and Shaffer, L. G. (2006). Application of array-based comparative genomic hybridization to clinical diagnostics, *J. Mol. Diagn.*, **8**(5), 528–33.

Beroukhim, R., et al. (2007), Assessing the significance of chromosomal aberrations in cancer: methodology and application to glioma, *Proc. Natl. Acad. Sci. USA*, **104**(50), 20007–12.

Bignell, G. R., et al. (2004), High-resolution analysis of DNA copy number using oligonucleotide microarrays, *Genome Res.*, **14**(2), 287–95.

Brennan, C., et al. (2004), High-resolution global profiling of genomic alterations with long oligonucleotide microarray, *Cancer Res.*, **64**(14), 4744–8.

Bruder, C. E., et al. (2008), Phenotypically concordant and discordant monozygotic twins display different DNA copy-number-variation profiles, *Am. J. Hum. Genet.*, **82**(3), 763–71.

Brunet, J. P., et al. (2004), Metagenes and molecular pattern discovery using matrix factorization, *Proc. Natl. Acad. Sci. USA*, **101**(12), 4164–9.

Campbell, P. J., et al. (2008), Identification of somatically acquired rearrangements in cancer using genome-wide massively parallel paired-end sequencing, *Nat. Genet.*, **40**(6), 722–9.

Cancer Genome Atlas Research Network (2008). Comprehensive genomic characterization defines human glioblastoma genes and core pathways. *Nature*, **23**;455 (7216), 1061–8.

Carrasco, D. R., et al. (2006), High-resolution genomic profiles defines distinct clinico-pathogenetic subgroups of multiple myeloma patients, *Cancer Cell*, **9**, 313–25.

Carter, N. P. (2007), Methods and strategies for analyzing copy number variation using DNA microarrays, *Nat. Genet.*, **39**(7 Suppl), S16–21.

Carvalho, B., et al. (2004), High resolution microarray comparative genomic hybridisation analysis using spotted oligonucleotides, *J. Clin. Pathol.*, **57**(6), 644–6.

Cheung, S. W., et al. (2005), Development and validation of a CGH microarray for clinical cytogenetic diagnosis, *Genet. Med.*, **7**(6), 422–32.

Cools, J., et al. (2003), A tyrosine kinase created by fusion of the PDGFRA and FIP1L1 genes as a therapeutic target of imatinib in idiopathic hypereosinophilic syndrome, *N. Engl. J. Med.*, **348**(13), 1201–14.

Diskin, S. J., et al. (2006), STAC: A method for testing the significance of DNA copy number aberrations across multiple array-CGH experiments, *Genome Res.*, **16**(9), 1149–58.

Engle, L. J., Simpson, C. L., and Landers, J. E. (2006), Using high-throughput SNP technologies to study cancer, *Oncogene*, **25**(11), 1594–601.

Ferguson, D. O., et al. (2000), The nonhomologous end-joining pathway of DNA repair is required for genomic stability and the suppression of translocations, *Proc. Natl. Acad. Sci. USA*, **97**(12), 6630–3.

Freeman, J. L., et al. (2006), Copy number variation: new insights in genome diversity, *Genome Res.*, **16**(8), 949–61.

Futreal, P. A., et al. (2004), A census of human cancer genes, *Nat. Rev. Cancer*, **4**(3), 177–83.

Greenman, C., et al. (2007), Patterns of somatic mutation in human cancer genomes, *Nature*, **446**(7132), 153–8.

Greshock, J., et al. (2007), A comparison of DNA copy number profiling platforms, *Cancer Res.*, **67**(21), 10173–80.

Guttman, M., et al. (2007), Assessing the significance of conserved genomic aberrations using high resolution genomic microarrays, *PLoS Genet.*, **3**(8), e143.

Hehir-Kwa, J. Y., et al. (2007), Genome-wide copy number profiling on high-density bacterial artificial chromosomes, single-nucleotide polymorphisms, and oligonucleotide microarrays: a platform comparison based on statistical power analysis, *DNA Res.*, **14**(1), 1–11.

Heiskanen, M. A., et al. (2000), Detection of gene amplification by genomic hybridization to cDNA microarrays, *Cancer Res.*, **60**(4), 799–802.

Hermans, K. G., et al. (2006), TMPRSS2:ERG fusion by translocation or interstitial deletion is highly relevant in androgen-dependent prostate cancer, but is bypassed in late-stage androgen receptor-negative prostate cancer, *Cancer Res.*, **66**(22), 10658–63.

Hsu, L., et al. (2005), Denoising array-based comparative genomic hybridization data using wavelets, *Biostatistics*, **6**(2), 211–26.

Hu, M., Yao, J., and Polyak, K. (2006), Methylation-specific digital karyotyping, *Nat. Protoc.*, **1**(3), 1621–36.

Hupe, P., et al. (2004), Analysis of array CGH data: from signal ratio to gain and loss of DNA regions, *Bioinformatics*, **20**(18), 3413–22.

Iafrate, A. J., et al. (2004), Detection of large-scale variation in the human genome, *Nat. Genet.*, **36**(9), 949–51.

Ishkanian, A. S., et al. (2004), A tiling resolution DNA microarray with complete coverage of the human genome, *Nat. Genet.*, **36**(3), 299–303.

Kallioniemi, A., et al. (1992), Comparative genomic hybridization for molecular cytogenetic analysis of solid tumors, *Science*, **258**(5083), 818–21.

Kennedy, G. C., et al. (2003), Large-scale genotyping of complex DNA, *Nat. Biotechnol.*, **21**(10), 1233–7.

Khaja, R., et al. (2006), Genome assembly comparison identifies structural variants in the human genome, *Nat. Genet.*, **38**(12), 1413–8.

Komura, D., et al. (2006), Noise reduction from genotyping microarrays using probe level information, *In Silico Biol.*, **6**(1–2), 79–92.

Korbel, J. O., et al. (2007), Systematic prediction and validation of breakpoints associated with copy-number variants in the human genome, *Proc. Natl. Acad. Sci. USA*, **104**(24), 10110–5.

Lai, W., Choudhary, V., and Park, P. J. (2008), CGHweb: a tool for comparing DNA copy number segmentations from multiple algorithms, *Bioinformatics*, **24**: 1014–1015.

Lai, W. R., et al. (2005), Comparative analysis of algorithms for identifying amplifications and deletions in array CGH data, *Bioinformatics*, **21**(19), 3763–70.

Liu, W., et al. (2007), Multiple genomic alterations on 21q22 predict various TMPRSS2/ERG fusion transcripts in human prostate cancers, *Genes Chromosomes Cancer*, **46**(11), 972–80.

Lucito, R., et al. (2003), Representational oligonucleotide microarray analysis: a high-resolution method to detect genome copy number variation, *Genome Res*, **13**(10), 2291–305.

Maher, E. A., et al. (2006), Marked genomic differences characterize primary and secondary glioblastoma subtypes and identify two distinct molecular and clinical secondary glioblastoma entities, *Cancer Res.*, **66**(23), 11502–13.

Marioni, J. C., Thorne, N. P., and Tavare, S. (2006), BioHMM: a heterogeneous hidden Markov model for segmenting array CGH data, *Bioinformatics*, **22**(9), 1144–6.

Olshen, A. B., et al. (2004), Circular binary segmentation for the analysis of array-based DNA copy number data, *Biostatistics*, **5**(4), 557–72.

Picard, F., et al. (2005), A statistical approach for array CGH data analysis, *BMC Bioinformatics*, **6**, 27.

Pinkel, D., et al. (1998), High resolution analysis of DNA copy number variation using comparative genomic hybridization to microarrays, *Nat. Genet.*, **20**(2), 207–11.

Pollack, J. R., et al. (1999), Genome-wide analysis of DNA copy-number changes using cDNA microarrays, *Nat. Genet.*, **23**(1), 41–6.

References

Redon, R., et al. (2006), Global variation in copy number in the human genome. *Nature*, **444**, 444–54.

Rigaill, G., et al. (2008), ITALICS: an algorithm for normalization and DNA copy number calling for Affymetrix SNP arrays, *Bioinformatics*, **24**(6), 768–74.

Sebat, J., et al. (2004). Large-scale copy number polymorphism in the human genome, *Science*, **305**(5683), 525–8.

Sharp, A. J., et al. (2007), Optimal design of oligonucleotide microarrays for measurement of DNA copy-number, *Hum. Mol. Genet.*, **16**(22), 2770–9.

—— (2005), Segmental duplications and copy-number variation in the human genome, *Am. J. Hum. Genet.*, **77**(1), 78–88.

Solinas-Toldo, S., et al. (1997), Matrix-based comparative genomic hybridization: biochips to screen for genomic imbalances, *Genes Chromosomes Cancer*, **20**(4), 399–407.

Solomon et al. (2008), Mutational inactivation of PTPRD in glioblastoma multiforme and malignant melanoma. *Cancer Res.*, **68**(24), 10300–6.

Stjernqvist, S., et al. (2007), Continuous-index hidden Markov modelling of array CGH copy number data, *Bioinformatics*, **23**(8), 1006–14.

Stranger, B. E., et al. (2007), Relative impact of nucleotide and copy number variation on gene expression phenotypes, *Science*, **315**(5813), 848–53.

Thorland, E. C., et al. (2007), Comprehensive validation of array comparative genomic hybridization platforms: how much is enough? *Genet. Med.*, **9**(9), 632–41.

Tonon, G., et al. (2005), High-resolution genomic profiles of human lung cancer, *Proc. Natl. Acad. Sci. USA*, **102**(27), 9625–30.

Venkatraman, E. S. and Olshen, A. B. (2007), A faster circular binary segmentation algorithm for the analysis of array CGH data, *Bioinformatics*, **23**(6), 657–63.

Xing, B., et al. (2007). A hierarchical clustering method for estimating copy number variation. *Biostatistics*, **8**(3), 632–53.

Wang, P., et al. (2005). A method for calling gains and losses in array CGH data. *Biostatistics*, **6**(1), 45–58.

Wang, T. L., et al. (2002), Digital karyotyping, *Proc. Natl. Acad. Sci. USA*, **99**(25), 16156–61.

Wang, Y., et al. (2007), Analysis of molecular inversion probe performance for allele copy number determination, *Genome Biol.*, **8**(11), R246.

Wiedemeyer, R., et al. (2008), Feedback circuit among INK4 tumour suppressors constrains human glioblastoma development, *Cancer Cell*, **13**(4), 355–64.

Wood, L. D., et al. (2007), The genomic landscapes of human breast and colorectal cancers, *Science*, **318**(5853), 1108–13.

3
METHODS FOR DERIVATION OF LOH AND ALLELIC COPY NUMBERS USING SNP ARRAYS

Carsten Wiuf, Philippe Lamy and Claus L. Andersen

3.1 Introduction

Genetic instability is a hallmark of most cancers and hence the cancer genome is often highly irregular. It is widely accepted that genetic instability is a key driver in the development and progression of cancer. With the advent of high-troughput technologies it has become possible to extensively investigate the genomic consequences of uncontrolled cell growth and tumourigenesis and to relate patterns of genetic changes to clinical outcomes, prognosis, and therapeutics. Whereas it previously was only possible to study single genes or small regions at a time, it is now possible to study the entire genome in a single experiment.

This chapter focuses on informatics methods to detect allelic imbalance (AI) and loss of heterozygozity (LOH) in particular. Here LOH refers only to the event that either the maternal or the paternal copy of a chromosomal region is deleted and not that a copy is functionally inactivated by mutation. LOH can be detected by comparing germline DNA with tumour DNA using genetic markers displaying

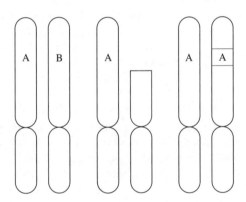

FIG. 3.1: The principle behind LOH analysis. The figure shows a heterozygous SNP on a pair of chromosomes in the germline DNA. If the part containing the B allele is deleted, then the remaining A allele will appear as a homozygous SNP. Likewise, if the B allele is converted following a recombination/gene conversion event, then the SNP will also appear homozygous. In the latter case there are two chromosomes present, while in the former there is only one for that particular SNP.

heterogeneity in the germline sample; see Fig. 3.1 for an example. However, if the marker is homozygous in the germline, it is non-informative about LOH and one cannot from that marker alone deduce whether LOH has occurred or not. AI, in contrast, refers generally to situations in which one allele is lost or amplified, and thus shows departure from the allelic copy number of the normal genome. In this terminology LOH is a special kind of AI.

The methods we are going to discuss are developed in the context of whole-genome Single Nucleotide Polymorphism (SNP) arrays which is a type of DNA microarray originally intended solely to genotype genetic polymorphisms within populations.

3.1.1 Overview

The following sections are built up such that we first discuss biological and historical aspects of LOH and AI. We discuss these aspects in the context of tumour supressor genes (TSGs) and retinoblastoma. Then we move on to discuss methods for derivation of LOH based on SNP array data, starting with some very simple methods that are often applied in the literature and end with discussing methods for derivation of AI based on hidden Markov models (HMMs). These models are popular tools in bioinformatics and frequently used to model dependencies in data sets (Durbin et al., 1998). We will give some examples to illustrate the methods.

3.1.2 Retinoblastoma

The concept of LOH is closely related to that of a TSG which is a gene that offers protection against an organismal cell transforming into a cancer cell. Probably the best known example of a TSG is the *RB1* gene that when inactivated causes retinoblastoma, cancer of the eye, which is a childhood disease. *RB1* is also the first TSG that was described in the literature and gave rise to Knudson's famous two-hit hypothesis from 1971 (Knudson, 1971).

Retinoblastoma occurs with an incidence of approximately 1 in 20,000 (Weinberg, 2007), results in clonal tumours in the retina and includes dominantly inherited as well as sporadic cases. The sporadic cases are often only present in a single focus in one eye, whereas the familiar cases typically involve both eyes and can be multifocal (Weinberg, 2007). Knudson compared the ages of children suffering from both forms of retinoblastoma and found that the sporadic cases generally occurred later in childhood than the familiar cases. This prompted Knudson to suggest the two-hit hypothesis – the hypothesis that two (genetic) hits are necessary for the cancer to develop. In the inherited cases the first hit occurs in the germline and the second in the target retinal cell, while in the sporadic cases both hits occur in the target retinal cell. This is consistent with the fact that the disease occurs earlier in childhood when inherited than when sporadic.

Cytogenetic studies identified chromosome 13 as a potential location of the harmful gene. Subsequent LOH analysis using Restriction Fragment Length Polymorphism (RFLP) markers (see Section 3.2) narrowed the relevant genomic region substantially until it was possible to pinpoint the exact gene *RB1* and its location in band 13q14. The *RB1* gene consists of 27 exons, spans 180kb and is known as a negative regulator of the cell cycle. According to the COSMIC data base at the Sanger Institute (2008) there are currently 75 known somatic substitutions in the *RB1*, 16 insertions and 43 deletions. These may all reduce expression of the *RB1* protein or disrupt translation completely. Only the deletions may turn up in an LOH analysis and in a patient suffering from retinoblastoma, the deletions are indicative of a second harmful mutation in the remaining copy of the *RB1* gene.

3.1.3 Identification of TSGs

TSGs are generally involved in cell cycle regulation or apoptosis, or both. Like *RB1* they are normally not haploinsufficient and a single copy of the gene is sufficient to produce the required amounts of gene product for the cell to be fully functioning.

TSG inactivation occurs in different ways as already described in the previous section. The most common inactivators are DNA point mutations, small insertions or deletions (few base pairs) or large deletions involving the whole TSG and potentially other genes. Since TSGs generally are not haplosufficient both copies of the gene must be inactivated before disruption of the gene function occurs – this reiterates the importance of Knudson's two-hit hypothesis. However, it also emphasizes that knowledge of TSGs and their function is key to understanding cancer progression and how cancer arises in the first place.

LOH analysis is central to pointing at genomic regions potentially harbouring novel TSGs, as illustrated in Fig. 3.1. Deletion of a region is the first indication that genes in the region may have reduced expression or have been functionally inactivated. The problem, however, is that LOH regions rarely cover just a single or few genes, but easily cover hundreds of genes. A subsequent mutational analysis is therefore not feasible, unless the analysis can be guided by other (functional) information about the genes.

3.1.4 Mechanisms causing AI (in particular LOH)

The molecular mechanism(s) responsible for creating AI are poorly understood. Studies of human cancers have indicated that most likely multiple mechanisms are involved. This is illustrated by the different types of LOH regions observed in human cancer; LOH of a whole chromosome, LOH extending from the telomere to involve the whole or part of a chromosome arm, and LOH at an interstitial chromosomal region. It is unlikely that these different types of regions are produced by the same mechanism. Until recently, LOH was considered to equal a reduced allelic (DNA) copy number. However, recent studies combining LOH and DNA copy number analyses have demonstrated that the DNA copy number of LOH regions can also be unaltered or even increased (Andersen *et al.*, 2007; Gaasenbeek *et al.*, 2006; Thiagalingam *et al.*, 2001). LOH regions with reduced copy number are said to be deleted, while regions with unaltered or increased copy numbers are said to display uniparental disomy or uniparental polysomy. Again, these observations indicate that multiple mechanisms are at play.

Several mechanisms have been suggested to cause LOH. Whole chromosome LOH may occur by 'non-disjunction' which refers to the situation, during mitosis, in which the duplicated chromosomes do not align properly. As a result the daughter cells end up with unequal chromosome numbers, one cell with three copies and the other with a single copy. In LOH and copy number analyses the latter daughter cell will display LOH and a reduced copy number of the whole chromosome. Whole chromosome LOH without reduced DNA copy number has been suggested to be the result of an non-disjunction event followed by a whole chromosome reduplication event.

Mitotic homologous recombination events could potentially result in telomeric and interstitial LOH regions (also called gene conversions). These events would be copy number neutral. However, telomeric and interstitial LOH regions often have a reduced DNA copy number, which indicates that other mechanisms are at play. These could be mitotic non-homologous recombination events, chromosomal breakage-fusion-bridge events (Gisselsson et al., 2000), or failures by the double-strand repair-recombination machinery (Ferguson et al., 2000).

3.1.5 Genomic alterations and their relation to clinical end-points

Many studies have demonstrated that genomic alterations observed in cancer are distributed in a non-random fashion across the genome (Weinberg, 2007). Whether the alterations initially occur at specific or random sites in the genome is presently not fully understood. However, it is a fact that natural selection drives tumour progression, i.e. the genomic alterations that benefit the survival and reproduction of the cancer cells in a tumour are the processes that drive the natural progression of the tumour, and also its ability to acquire resistance to therapy (Merlo et al., 2006). Hence, non-random alterations observed in the cancer genome pinpoint regions likely to be of importance for the survival and reproduction of cancer cells. LOH involving chromosome band 17p13.1 inactivating the tumour suppressor gene TP53 (thereby, improving the survival of cancer cells) is a classical example of a non-random alteration occurring at high frequency in many different cancer types. Evidently, alterations affecting specific genes infer specific phenotypic traits to the tumour, i.e. resistance to growth inhibition, evasion of apoptosis, angiogenesis, invasion, and metastasis (Vogelstein and Kinzler, 2004). It has been argued that a limited number of alterations is necessary to transform a normal cell into a neoplastic cell and that the order in which these alterations occur is stochastic (Hanahan and Weinberg, 2000).

This led to the hypothesis that differences in the genetic makeup of histopathologically similar tumours may be responsible for differences observed in prognosis and treatment response. Along this line several studies have investigated the potential of using genomic alterations (LOH) as prognostic biomarkers. A retrospective study of 467 Multiple Myeloma cases showed that LOH at chromosome arm 16q conferred a poor prognosis (Jenner et al., 2007). Similarly, a retrospective study of 106 curatively resected colorectal cancers showed that LOH at chromosome arm 18q is associated with an increased risk of both local and distant recurrence of disease (Sarli et al., 2004). Another retrospective study of 460 stage III and high risk stage II colon cancer patients treated adjuvantly with fluorouracil also indicated that 18q LOH is associated with poor outcome (Watanabe et al., 2001).

LOH markers have also been investigated in relation to prediction of treatment response. A retrospective study of 149 patients diagnosed with Glioma and treated with temozolomide showed that LOH at chromosome arms 1p and 19q predicted both a durable chemosensitivity and a favourable outcome (Kaloshi et al., 2007).

Currently, prospective clinical trials are being performed aiming to transfer promising molecular biomarkers, including LOH markers, from the research setting to clinical decision making. An example of this is the large E5202 trial of the Eastern Cooperative Oncology Group which is evaluating the use of 18q LOH to guide the choice of whether or not to apply adjuvant chemotherapy to stage II colon cancer patients (http://www.cancer.gov/clinicaltrials/ECOG-E5202).

3.2 Experimental determination of LOH

Most experimental methods for genotyping are qualitative in the sense that they only allow determination of the presence or the absence of an allele.[1] Without the possibility to measure absolute genomic quantities, LOH can only be derived by comparing germline DNA with tumour DNA. For example, if the germline of a particular marker is heterozygous (AB), but only one of the two alleles is observed in the tumour sample then LOH can be inferred. One of the two alleles must have been lost and the genotype in the tumour will appear as either AA or BB.

Therefore, only markers heterozygous in the germline are informative about the LOH status of the corresponding markers in the tumour tissue. Consequently, multi-allelic markers should be preferred to bi-allelic markers, because the chance that a multi-allelic marker is heterozygous is generally higher than the chance that a bi-allelic marker is. Traditionally, microsatellite markers have been applied because they show a plethora of alleles varying in length, but also RFLP markers have been used, because of their greater abundance in the genome. RFLP markers are bi-allelic markers showing the absence (−) or presence (+) of a restriction enzyme cut-point.

The large-scale discovery of bi-allelic SNPs and the advent of SNP microarray technologies have by far made SNP the preferred marker for LOH and copy number studies. The HapMap project (http://www.hapmap.org/) lists over 5 million validated SNPs in the human genome, or more than one in 600 base pairs. For

---

[1]This remark is only true if we look at markers one by one. We shall later discuss how these restrictions can be relaxed when using microarrays with many markers. It is possible quantitatively to derive the copy numbers and hence also the LOH status of homozygous markers.

whole genome-scans or high-resolution maps of LOH, SNPs are therefore today the natural choice. Generally, bi-allelic markers suffer from lack of information because the fraction of individuals in a population heterozygous for a given marker is always less than 50%, and consequently at most half of the markers are informative about LOH. However, this lack of information is counterbalanced by the very high number of known SNPs and their very high density in the genome.

3.3 SNP genotyping arrays

The first SNP genotyping arrays to be marketed were Affymetrix SNP arrays in 1994. They targeted 1500 SNPs in the human genome. Since then many larger arrays have been commercialized (http://www.affymetrix.com) and many other companies have entered the scene, e.g. Illumina Inc. The newest versions of Affymetrix and Illumina arrays host ~1 million SNPs. The array quality has increased largely over the years due to technological and experimental advances.

In the following we focus on Affymetrix SNP arrays. Each SNP is represented by a series of probes. The probes are of two kinds: mismatch (MM) and perfect match (PM) probes, and these are made specific to the two alleles. A PM probe is typically around 20 nucleotides long and matches one of the alleles and the surrounding nucleotides perfectly. By moving the position of the SNP in the probe, one gets a series of allele specific PM probes with different binding affinities. The MM probes are similar, but the centre position in the probe does not match the reference sequence. The idea is that MM probes measure non-specific binding, but it has been debated widely to what extent the information obtained from MM probes is useful for genotype and copy number inference. Most statistical approaches applied to SNP arrays ignore MM probes. There are up to 20 PM probes for each allele.

By nature of the experimental set-up and measurements it is not possible to detect ploidy differences, i.e. one cannot distinguish between a genome with two copies of each chromosome and a genome with e.g. four copies.

3.3.1 *Normalization*

The probe intensities must be normalized before they can be applied to address biological questions (Carvalho *et al.*, 2007; Draghici, 2003; Speed, 2003). Firstly, intensities between arrays are not directly comparable because the total amount of DNA in samples varies and secondly, the relationship between array intensities need not be linear. These issues are common to microarrays in general and we will not be concerned with the details here, but refer to the large literature available on the subject (Speed, 2003; Carvalho *et al.*, 2007). For Affymetrix SNP arrays the standard has become to use the *invariant set* normalization procedure advocated by Li and Wong (2001) and implemented in the dChipSNP software package. This procedure selects a core set of probe intensities that are used for calibration of intensity levels. Subsequently, the probe intensities for a particular SNP are combined into a single variable, or two variables, if the intensities are kept separately for the two alleles.

Here we apply a simple average to describe the allele intensity as a single variable

$$I_A = \frac{1}{p} \sum_{i=1}^{p} \log(\text{PM}_i(A)), \tag{3.1}$$

where $\text{PM}_i(A)$ denotes the intensity of the ith PM probe for allele A. A similar quantity is calculated for allele B.

The allele intensities are now comparable across arrays, but not necessarily between neighbouring SNPs on the same array, because the chemical binding properties of the probes depend on the DNA sequence – this is an important issue that must be dealt with in order to conduct LOH analysis properly. We will take the issue up in Section 3.6.

3.3.2 Genotyping

Generally, the absence of an intensity signal of a given allele, potentially measured relatively to a reference, indicates the absence of that allele in the genotype. In a normal sample where all autosomal markers are assumed to exist in two copies, the presence/absence of alleles is sufficient to determine the genotype completely including the number of each allele: AA (presence of A, absence of B), AB (presence of A and B), and BB (absence of A, presence of B). For chromosome X markers presence/absence of alleles is also sufficient to determine the genotype, if it is known whether the sample is from a male or female (otherwise one cannot distinguish between, e.g. AY and AA). Naturally, for abnormal samples it is not possible to infer the genotype from the presence and absence of alleles only, as has already been discussed in Section 3.2. In recent years it has become apparent that many loci in the genome show copy number variations that are inherited in a Mendelian fashion. Known copy number variations (mainly detected with SNP arrays, Redon et al., 2006, White et al., 2007) are still relatively few and we will ignore them here.

However, the intensity signals carry information about the copy number of a particular allele. In several studies it has been demonstrated that the logarithm of the intensity is proportional to the logarithm of the allelic copy number; as demonstrated in Fig. 3.2. This relationship is true even for very high copy numbers.

In Fig. 3.3, five clouds are easily distinguishable, one for each of the possible genotypes of a chromosome X marker. There are two important observations to be made from Figs. 3.2 and 3.3: The first is that the log-intensity log-copy number relationship does not hold if there are zero copies, because of background and non-specific binding that elevate the intensity level from the expected level. The log-copy number would be large and negative, if the hypothesis were true (log(0) is minus infinity). The second is that we would expect the same

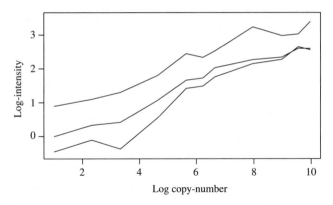

FIG. 3.2: The relationship between log-intensity and log-copy number. The figure shows three (out of 42) SNPs in a spiking experiment where the concentration (copy number) of each SNP is varied from 1 to 1000 (Bignell et al., 2004). Clearly there is a linear relationship between the log-intensity and the log-copy number. Each data point is based on one measurement, occasionally on two.

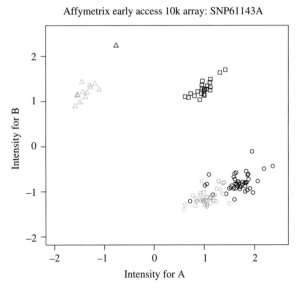

FIG. 3.3: Allele intensities in normal tissue. The figure shows allele intensities, as defined in eqn (3.1) from one SNP located on chromosome X (SNP61143A from an Affymetrix array) in a sample of 67 males and 57 females. The genotypes AA (black circle), AB (black square), BB (black triangle), AX (grey circle) and BX (grey triangle) are clearly distinguishable. Note that the A intensity for the BB and BX genotypes is elevated due to non-specific binding and background, corresponding to approximately 0.25 copies of the A allele. (The same is true for the B intensity of the AA and AX genotypes.)

difference in intensity between 1 and 2 copies, as between 2 and 4, and in general between 2^n and 2^{n+1} copies, because $\log_2(2^{n+1}) - \log_2(2^n) = 1$ for all n. This naturally implies that it is much more difficult statistically to distinguish between 3 and 4 copies ($\log_2(4) - \log_2(3) \approx 0.42$) than between 1 and 2 copies ($\log_2(2) - \log_2(1) = 1$).

3.4 Simple computational tools to infer LOH

3.4.1 Classification of genotypes

Assuming the genotype status of each marker can be determined without error, then loss of heterozygosity or retention can be inferred without error for each heterozygous marker. For homogeneous markers, LOH inference is only possible in conjunction with neighbouring markers, as will be demonstrated below. Genotypes are recorded as AA, AB, BB, or NC (No Call), irrespective of the number of actual copies of a given allele in the tissue. AB is said to be informative, while the remaining genotypes (AA, BB, and NC) are said to be non-informative. For informative markers, LOH status is either loss (L) or retention (R); for non-informative markers, loss (L), retention (R), or undecided (U). LOH status L and R are said to be proper LOH status, and U is said to be improper.

3.4.2 Regions with same boundary (RSB)

Consider the example in Fig. 3.4 with six bi-allelic markers, three of which are informative, i.e. they are heterozygous in the germline sample. There are various simple computational tools to infer the LOH status of non-informative markers. The methods are simple extensions of the immediate classification of markers according to whether the observed genotypes are indicative of loss or not. We will mention two methods here; both methods are based on the principle of parsimony which states that if two explanations are possible one should choose the explanation that in some sense is the most parsimonious or the simplest. In the RSB method, LOH status is first inferred for all informative markers. In Fig. 3.4 there are only three informative markers (1, 4, and 6). Markers 4, 6 are indicative of LOH, while marker 1 indicates retention. The LOH status of a non-informative marker bounded by two informative markers is assigned according to the status of the two informative markers. If the bounding markers agree, then

```
Germline  AB  AA  AA  AB  AA  AB
Tumour    AB  AA  AA  AA  AA  AA
```

FIG. 3.4: An example illustrating simple computational tools to infer LOH. The figure shows six markers, but only three are heterozygous in the germline and thus informative about LOH. The RSB method assigns L to marker 5, while markers 2 and 3 are U because they are surrounded by an R and an L. Thus, the six markers have status RUULLL. The NN method assigns L to markers 3 and 5, and R to marker 2; that is, the six markers have status RRLLLL.

the non-informative markers obtain the same status as the informative markers, but if the bounding markers do not agree, the status is left undecided. In the figure, marker 5 shows loss, while markers 2 and 3 are undecided. Using this method, some markers may end up being undecided. This happens whenever a non-informative marker is bounded by two informative makers with opposite status, as is the case for markers 1 and 4.

3.4.3 Nearest Neighbour (NN)

The NN method differs from the RSB method. In the NN method, the LOH status of a non-informative marker is determined from the nearest informative marker. In Fig. 3.4 this implies that the status of marker 2 is retention, that of marker 3 is loss and that of marker 5 is loss. This method implies that all markers receive a LOH status, unless there are no informative markers at all, in which case there would be no nearest neighbours. Whenever the RSB method assigns a proper status, the same status is assigned by NN – however, the reverse is not true as is illustrated in Fig. 3.4.

3.5 Advanced statistical tools for LOH inference

The simple tools to infer LOH status are too simple in several ways. In the present formulation they are not able to handle missing data or errors in the reported genotypes, and the assignment of LOH status is purely deterministic relying only on the nearest informative markers. Furthermore, some markers may end up with an improper status. This is naturally not satisfactory in many situations. Missing data could be handled by introducing additional rules, e.g. if the genotype in the germline sample is missing, but heterozygous in the tumour sample then retention is assigned, and so forth; or all missing genotypes could be termed undecided. However, these issues are more naturally dealt with in a probabilistic or statistical set-up and several have been proposed in the literature. Here we will only deal with one general framework.

3.5.1 Hidden Markov models

Hidden Markov models (HMMs) have been shown to be a useful tool for LOH and copy number inference (Fridlyand et al., 2004; Lin et al., 2004; Koed et al., 2005) and one such approach has been implemented in the well-known software package, dChipSNP, for SNP array analysis. HMMs are probabilistic models that are able to take correlations in the data into account and use this information to guide the inference when data are sparse or missing.

The concept of a HMM is explained in Fig. 3.5 and Table 3.1. Underlying the observations are *hidden states* (in our case loss or retention; but not undecided); we only observe the hidden states indirectly through the observed genotypes. Each marker is either in the loss state or in the retention state. If a marker is in the loss state, only certain genotype combinations in the germline and the tumour samples are possible and with certain probabilities; and similarly if in the retention state (see Section 3.5.2 for an example). Because markers close

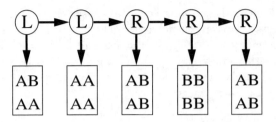

FIG. 3.5: An example of a hidden Markov model (HMM). The top row shows the genomic states, L or R, of the abnormal sample. When in state L, the HMM stays in the same state with probability p and jumps to the state R with probability $1-p$, see Table 3.1. If p is small, deleted segments are small, while they are longer if p is large. Likewise, when in state R, the HMM stays in the same state with probability q and jumps to the state L with probability $1-q$ (p and q need not be identical). If q is large there will be few deleted segments (few jumps from R to L), while there will be more if q is small. The state determines which genotype combinations are possible and with which probabilities. If there are no call errors in the data, then AB-AA is only possible in the L state; however if call errors are allowed then AB-AA could also be emitted in the R state.

TABLE 3.1. Shown are the probabilities of going from state $S_{i-1} = L$ or $S_{i-1} = R$ of marker $i-1$ to state $S_i = L$ or $S_i = R$ of marker i.

Marker $i-1$	Marker i L	R
L	p	$1-p$
R	$1-q$	q

to each other are likely to share LOH status, the hidden states are modelled through a dependency structure, called a Markov chain.

Let S_i (= L, or R) be the hidden state of marker i, where $i = 1, \ldots, k$ (e.g. $k = 50{,}000$) and the markers are ordered according to their physical position along the chromosome. The Markov property dictates that the probability of being in states $S_1, S_2, \ldots, S_k$ is given by

$$P(S_1, S_2, \ldots, S_k) = P(S_1)P(S_2|S_1) \cdots P(S_k|S_{k-1}) \qquad (3.2)$$

such that the probability is split into a product of k terms. The term $P(S_i|S_{i-1})$ is the probability that marker i is in state S_i given the state of the neighbour marker. Since there are two possibilities for S_i and two for S_{i-1}, there are four in total and the probabilities of these can be given in the form of a table; see Table 3.1.

The parameters p and q in Table 3.1 are unknown and describe how likely it is that a deleted (or retained) region is extended by an extra marker. Likewise the probability of the first marker being L or R depends on p and q only,

$$P(\text{L}) = \frac{1-q}{2-p-q} \quad \text{and} \quad P(\text{R}) = 1 - P(\text{L}) = \frac{1-p}{2-p-q}. \qquad (3.3)$$

For example if $p = 0.7$ and $q = 0.9$, then the probability of RRRLLRL is

$$\frac{1-0.7}{2-0.7-0.9} \cdot 0.9 \cdot 0.9 \cdot (1-0.9) \cdot 0.7 \cdot (1-0.7) \cdot (1-0.9) = 1.28 \cdot 10^{-3},$$

where each term (apart from the first) corresponds to a transition from one marker to the next.

The likelihood $L(G_1, G_2, \ldots, G_k)$ of a set of paired germline-tumour genotype observations (as in Fig. 3.4 with six paired genotypes) can be calculated as

$$\begin{aligned}
L(G_1, \ldots, G_k) &= \sum_{S_1, \ldots, S_k} P(G_1, \ldots, G_k | S_1, \ldots, S_k) P(S_1, \ldots, S_k) \\
&= \sum_{S_1, S_2, \ldots, S_k} P(G_1|S_1) P(G_2|S_2) \cdots P(G_k|S_k) P(S_1, S_2, \ldots S_k),
\end{aligned} \qquad (3.4)$$

where $S_1, S_2, \ldots, S_k$ are the hidden states and the sum is over all possible combinations of hidden states; i.e. for each combination of hidden states a probability is assigned to the observed genotypes. When the hidden states are given we assume the genotypes are independent of each other, hence $P(G_1, \ldots, G_k | S_1, \ldots, S_k)$ splits into a product with one term for each marker. Some combinations may be very unlikely (for example frequent jumps between loss and retention), and some combinations might render the observed genotypes very unlikely or impossible, e.g. the genotypes in Fig. 3.4 would have low probability if all hidden states are retention, because the first genotype is indicative of loss.

3.5.2 Example

There are various ways one can relate the hidden states to the genotypes; one example is given in Table 3.2. Each of the pairs is emitted with a certain probability. In this example we assume that the genotypes are measured without error and hence AB-AB can only occur in the R state and not in the L state. Also, the probability of being heterozygous in the germline is the same irrespective of the state of the tumour, namely r.

TABLE 3.2. Here it is assumed that genotyping errors are impossible, and thus the probability of emitting AB-AA in state R is zero, likewise the probability of emitting AB-AB is zero in state L. The parameter r is effectively the fraction of heterozygous SNPs in the germline DNA.

Hidden State	Genotype Pairs				
	AA-AA	BB-BB	AB-AB	AB-AA	AB-BB
L	$\frac{1}{2}(1-r)$	$\frac{1}{2}(1-r)$	0	$\frac{1}{2}r$	$\frac{1}{2}r$
R	$\frac{1}{2}(1-r)$	$\frac{1}{2}(1-r)$	r	0	0

TABLE 3.3. Shown are the combinations of hidden states with non-zero probabilities. In total there are 32, but the remaining combinations have probability zero, because they are incompatible with R in position 1, L in position 4 or L in position 6. In this example the probabilities P(Genotypes|States) end up being the same, because emitting AA-AA (BB-BB) has the same probability in the states L and R.

States	P(States)	P(Genotypes|States)
RRRLLL	$2.98 \cdot 10^{-2}$	$2.89 \cdot 10^{-4}$
RRLLLL	$2.32 \cdot 10^{-2}$	$2.89 \cdot 10^{-4}$
RLLLLL	$1.80 \cdot 10^{-2}$	$2.89 \cdot 10^{-4}$
RLRLLL	$1.10 \cdot 10^{-3}$	$2.89 \cdot 10^{-4}$
RRRLRL	$1.82 \cdot 10^{-3}$	$2.89 \cdot 10^{-4}$
RRLLRL	$1.41 \cdot 10^{-3}$	$2.89 \cdot 10^{-4}$
RLLLRL	$1.10 \cdot 10^{-3}$	$2.89 \cdot 10^{-4}$
RLRLRL	$6.75 \cdot 10^{-5}$	$2.89 \cdot 10^{-4}$

If we continue the example of six markers in Fig. 3.4, we note that the RSB method gives the RUULLL, while NN gives RRLLLL. In the HMM there are many possible assignments of states and they occur with different probabilities. In Table 3.3 we assume $p = 0.7$, $q = 0.9$ and $r = 0.3$ (which roughly corresponds to the percentage of heterozygous SNPs in Affymetrix arrays). The best scoring assignment is different from the one obtained using NN.

One strength of the HMM approach is that errors can be allowed leading to more correct inference (Lin et al., 2004; Koed et al., 2005).

3.5.3 Two main problems

There are two main problems we need to tackle:
- For a fixed set of parameters, determination of the optimal choice of hidden states, i.e. the assignment of hidden states contributing most to the likelihood. In Example 3.5.2 the optimal assignment is RRRLLL.
- Determination of the optimal choice of the HMM parameters (in Example 3.5.2, p and q) and the emitting probabilites (in Example 3.5.2, only r). In Example 3.5.2 the parameters were fixed, but in general they are unknown and should be estimated from the data.

Both problems can be solved with efficient algorithms and we will not go further into the issue here.

3.5.4 An interpretation of the hidden Markov model

Using HMMs for analysis of biological data, in particular DNA sequence data or data that are presented in a sequential order, is commonplace (Durbin et al., 1998). In addition to being very flexible and robust modelling tools, HMMs are computationally and statistically easy to manipulate.

However, the HMM also stipulates a mathematical model of the data, in our case loss of heterozygosity in tumours. The proportion of SNPs in the LOH state is $(1-q)/(2-p-q)$, see eqn (3.3), while the remaining SNPs are in the retention state. We can also derive the probability distribution of the length of a LOH region,

$$P(n) = (1-p)p^{n-1}, \qquad (3.5)$$

where p is the probability given in Table 3.1 and $n \geq 1$ is the number of SNPs in the LOH region. This distribution is known as the geometric distribution with parameter p and a LOH region has an expected length of $1/(1-p)$ SNPs. With the parameters of Example 3.5.2 this would amount only to $1/0.3 \approx 3.3$ SNPs. Likewise, the length of a retained region is geometric with parameter q resulting in an expected length of $1/(1-q) = 1/0.1 = 10$ SNPs. In this example LOH regions and retained regions are interchanged frequently.

A similar model has been applied to analyse cytogenetic data (Newton and Lee, 2000). Also a HMM approach has been suggested for the analysis of CGH array data (Fridlyand et al., 2004).

3.5.5 Limitations to the HMM approach

The HMM approach has a number of limitations. We assume two different states only, loss and retention, but in some cases it can be difficult to assign a single state to a genomic region. Sample heterogeneity may cause the copy number to be non-integer, for example if a fraction of the tumour cells have lost the region while other tumour cells have not, or if the size of the region varies between tumour cells. Also sample impurities may result in non-integer copy number. This may

(a) Normal

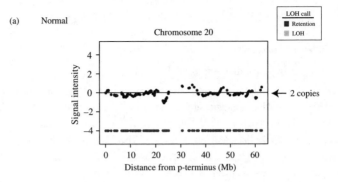

(b) Loss of the p-arm and gain of the q-arm

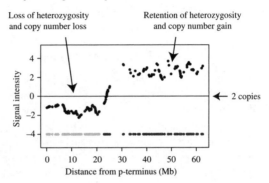

(c) Loss of the p-arm and uniparental polysomy of the q-arm

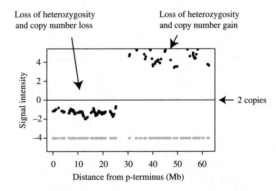

FIG. 3.6: The figure shows LOH and log-intensity data from three colon cancer patients using Affymetrix 10K SNP arrays. For each of the three patients array data were obtained from germline and tumour tissue. The dChipSNP software package was used to derive LOH based on a HMM that takes NC and genotyping errors into account. Also copy number intensities (joint for both alleles) were derived with dChipSNP software and further normalized to mean zero and variance one. The three parts of the figure show chromosome 20 in the tumour sample from the three patients. (a) LOH and copy numbers are normal, (b) factual loss of p-arm (i.e. LOH concomitant with copy number reduction) and gain of q-arm (i.e. retention of both alleles and simultaneous copy number increase), (c) factual loss of the p-arm and uniparental polysomy of the q-arm (i.e. LOH and concomitant copy number increase of the remaining allele).

TABLE 3.4. Shown are summary statistics from 17 patients with bladder cancer genotyped with the Affymetrix 10k array. In total 43 tumour samples were available (2–3 samples from each patient). Ta, T1 and T2-4 are different progressive stages of the disease and the numbers confirm that the genome becomes more instable with more progressed disease stage: The number of heterozygous SNPs decreases while the number of homozygous SNPs increases with stage, indicating that the progressed samples have more deletions than the less progressed samples. Also, the number of NCs increases with stage in concordance with the discussion in Section 3.5.5. The same conclusions hold for newer and larger Affymetrix arrays, as well as Illumina arrays.

	Blood	Ta	T1	T2-4
Heterozygous SNPs	2,721 (31%)	2,520 (29%)	2,156 (25%)	1,829 (21%)
Homozygous SNPs	5,648 (65%)	5,692 (66%)	5,878 (68%)	6,057 (70%)
No Call (NC)	317 (4%)	474 (5%)	652 (7%)	800 (9%)

occur, if the pathologist has not been succesful in removing surrounding normal tissue, or if the tumour sample naturally consists of cancer cells mixed with normal cells.

Another possibility is that one allele has been lost while the other has been duplicated to restore two copies (uniparental disomy; see Section 3.1.4). Thereby the functional integrity of a gene in the region may be intact unless one or both copies of the duplicated gene have been inactivated by other means. In the HMM approach, this event cannot be distinguished from the event of loss of one allele and maintainance of the other allele in one copy, because in both situations the HMM readout is a transition from AB in the germline to AA or BB in the tumour (or for homozygous SNPs AA or BB in the germline to AA og BB in the tumour) This is illustrated in Fig. 3.6.

As seen in Table 3.4 the number of NC is generally higher in tumour samples than in samples from normal tissue. This may partly be explained by heterogeneity and tissue impurities, because fractional copy numbers may be difficult to interpret correctly. In dChipSNP software (Lin et al., 2004), NCs in tumour samples are given no special status compared to normal samples, while the higher number of NCs was taken as evidence of LOH in Koed et al. (2005). However, NCs may also appear, if one or both alleles have been amplified resulting in distortions of the intensity values.

3.6 Estimation of allele specific copy numbers

In this section we discuss a HMM for estimation of allele specific copy numbers. The primary concern is *not* to derive genomic copy numbers, but to be able to investigate the allelic composition of genomic regions. Naturally, if we know the copy number of the two alleles, the genomic copy number can be determined by adding the two allele specific copy numbers – however the HMM has inherited limitations of a combinatorial as well as a statistical nature that makes it difficult to disentangle the allele specific copy numbers when the genomic copy number is high. This HMM approach is developed by Lamy et al. (2007) – other approaches to allele specific copy number derivation have been developed by Nannya et al. (2005), Huang et al. (2006), LaFramboise et al. (2005) and Ishikawa et al. (2006), but none of them use HMMs directly.

3.6.1 An allele specific HMM

The first part is to determine the HMM states. Since we want to infer the copy number of each allele, we need more than the genotypes determined from the germline and tumour samples: The genotypes could only tell whether an allele was retained or lost, not whether an allele was amplified.

Therefore, we need to work directly with the allele intensities, since these reflect the underlying copy numbers; as illustrated in Figs. 3.2 and 3.3. This further implies that the probability, $P(G|S)$ of a genotype G given the genomic state S of the tumour should be replaced by the density $f(I_A, I_B|S)$ of the two allele intensities given the state S. The density is here conveniently taken to be normal. The normal density has two mean parameters (one for I_A and one for I_B) and a covariance matrix with three parameters (the variances of I_A and I_B, and their correlation). This results in five parameters for each state and SNP. With thousands of SNPs and generally much fewer samples the number of parameters quickly becomes statistically unmanageable.

To resolve the hurdle, we rely on two main assumptions (Lamy et al., 2007): The first is the already mentioned linear relationship between log-intensity and log-copy number that binds the mean parameters of different states together. The second assumption states that the mean parameters of different SNPs are also related in a linear fashion; see Fig. 3.7. We note that other authors have solved the many-parameter problem in other ways; see for example Rabbee and Speed (2006) for a Bayesian solution in the context of SNP genotyping. In practice, we exclude SNPs that do not fit the assumption of linearity.

3.6.2 Normalization

There is a clear linear relationship between intensities and copy numbers, as illustrated in Fig. 3.7. We utilize this feature to normalize the data (Lamy et al., 2006). For the ith SNP (e.g. $i = 1, \ldots, 50,000$) and jth allele ($j =$ A, B) assume

$$\log_2(M_{ij}^2) = k_1 + k_2 \log_2(M_{ij}^1), \tag{3.6}$$

where M_{ij}^2 is the mean intensity for allele j in samples homozygous for the j allele, M_{ij}^1 is the mean intensity for allele j in samples heterozygous for the j allele, and k_1 and k_2 are SNP-independent parameters.

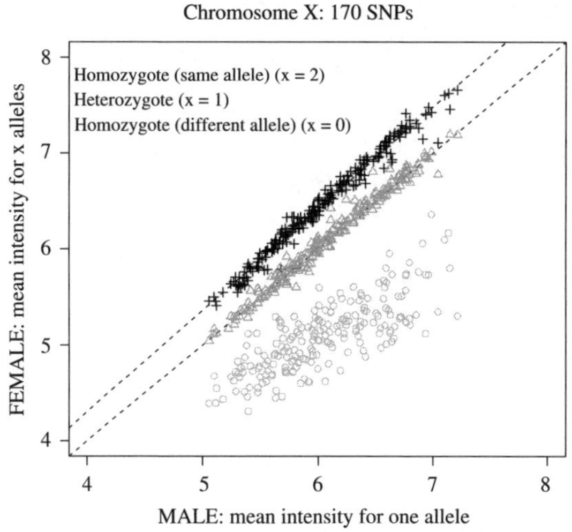

Chromosome X: 170 SNPs

Homozygote (same allele) (x = 2)
Heterozygote (x = 1)
Homozygote (different allele) (x = 0)

FEMALE: mean intensity for x alleles vs. MALE: mean intensity for one allele

FIG. 3.7: 170 chromosome X SNPs are used from a sample of 57 normal males and 67 normal females. For each allele the average is taken over all males with that particular allele and plotted against the average intensity of females with 0, 1 and 2 copies, respectively.

If we further assume that the logarithm of the allele copy number is linearly related to the log-intensity, then

$$\log_2(C_{ij}) = a_i + b_i \log_2(M_{ij}^c), \tag{3.7}$$

where C_{ij} is the allelic copy number and M_{ij}^c is the mean intensity of allele j in SNP i, respectively. The parameters a_i and b_i are SNP-specific. Here we let C_{ij} be an arbitrary number to allow for mixed samples.

From eqns (3.6) and (3.7) we find C_{ij} in term of M_{ij}^1 and M_{ij}^c:

$$\log_2(C_{ij}) = \frac{\log_2(M_{ij}^c) - \log_2(M_{ij}^1)}{k_1 + (k_2 - 1)\log_2(M_{ij}^1)}. \tag{3.8}$$

This equation remains true even if C_{ij} is not an integer.

As we only have the intensity I_{ij} of SNP i and allele j, an estimate of M_{ij}^c, we can only obtain X_{ij}, an estimate of $\log_2(C_{ij})$; i.e.

$$X_{ij}^c = \frac{\log_2(I_{ij}) - \log_2(M_{ij}^1)}{k_1 + (k_2 - 1)\log_2(M_{ij}^1)}. \tag{3.9}$$

We assume that X_{ij} is normally distributed around $\log(C_{ij})$ with (known) standard deviation estimated from the germline samples. Likewise, the parameters k_1 and k_2, as well as M_{ij}^1, are estimated from the germline samples.

3.6.3 The states

In the HMM there are six states for heterozygous SNPs and a corresponding number of states for homozygous SNPs (Fig. 3.8). Since it is difficult to distinguish between higher copy numbers, the HMM focuses on differentiating low copy numbers and lumps all larger copy numbers into one state. For heterozygous SNPs, the states indicate retention of both alleles, loss of one or both alleles, gain of one or both, and loss of one and gain of the other. These are clearly distinguishable states, since in each case we expect 0, 1 or 2 (or more) copies of a given allele (Fig. 3.8). The states of the homozygous SNPs are made to match those of the heterozygous SNPs. This is not straigthforward. For example the homozygous state corresponding to the heterozygous state (1,2+) is (0,3+) (Fig. 3.8), and the homozygous state corresponding to the heterozygous state (0,2+) is (0,2+). While each heterozygous SNP is classified to a unique state, a homozygous SNP may be classified to one or more states. A homozygous SNP with four B alleles could for example be assigned to (0,3+) as well as to (0,2+), but whether it is assigned to one state or the other depends to some extent on the surrounding heterozygous SNPs.

The parameters for going from one state to the next are also more elaborate now than for the previous HMM. In the previous HMM, one could go from R to L or from L to R. Inclusion of a gain state and differentiation between alleles make many more transitions possible, and we need to decide what is considered biologically realistic or plausible. Here we only consider transitions between states that require a single change, e.g. amplification of one allele. Further, we distinguish between going from (or to) the normal state, and going between two abnormal states.

This puts us in a situation to calculate the likelihoood of the observed intensities in a tumour sample, similarly to eqn (3.4):

$$L(I_{1A}, I_{1B}, \ldots, I_{kA}, I_{kB})$$
$$= \sum_{S_1, S_2, \ldots, S_k} f(I_{1A}, I_{1B}|S_1) \cdots f(I_{kA}, I_{kB}|S_k) P(S_1, S_2, \ldots, S_k), \quad (3.10)$$

where $f(I_{iA}, I_{iB}|S_i)$ denotes a normal distribution with mean determined by the state S_i. As pointed out in Section 3.5.3, there are efficient algorithms to optimize the unknown parameters (Fig. 3.8c) and to find the optimal choice of hidden states (Fig. 3.8a). Also for each SNP one can derive the probability that the HMM is in a given state.

3.6.4 Example

We ran the HMM on paired samples (tumour and blood) from 21 patients suffering from bladder cancer using intensities derived from Affymetrix 50k arrays (Lamy et al., 2007; Zieger et al., 2005). Not all SNPs were used, but only SNPs that were classifed as 'normal' (i.e. total copy number two) in the blood samples were selected for further analysis. This was accomplished by first running

Estimation of allele specific copy numbers 71

(a)

State	DNA copy-number	(A,B) N = AB	(A,B) N = AA	(A,B) N = BB
0	2	(1,1)	(2,0)	(0,2)
1	1	(0,1) or (1,0)	(1,0)	(0,1)
2	0	(0,0)	(0,0)	(0,0)
3	2+	(0,2+) or (2+,0)	(2+,0)	(0,2+)
4	3+	(1,2+) or (2+,1)	(3+,0)	(0,3+)
5	4+	(2+,2+)	(4+,0)	(0,4+)

(c)

State	1	2	3	4	5
0	p	p	ε	p	p
1		r	r	ε	ε
2			ε	ε	ε
3				r	r
4					r

(b)

STATE 0

STATE 1

STATE 2

STATE 3

STATE 4

STATE 5

(d)

$p : 0 \to 1$

$r : 1 \to 2$

$\varepsilon : 0 \to 3$

$0 \to 5$

$3 \to 4$

$2 \to 4$

FIG. 3.8: States and transition matrix of the HMM. (a) This figure shows the definition of the states in the HMM. The genotype call for the germline DNA is given by the letter N = AB, AA or BB. For each state, the total DNA copy number and the allelic copy numbers are given. State 0 is the germline state also called the normal state; state 1 corresponds to a heterozygous deletion (loss of one allele); state 2 corresponds to a homozygous deletion (loss of two alleles); state 3 corresponds to uniparental di/polysomy (loss of one allele and duplication or multiplication of the other allele); state 4 corresponds to unbalanced amplification (duplication or multiplication of only one allele); state 5 corresponds to balanced amplification (duplication or multiplication of both alleles). Notice that when the SNP marker in the germline DNA is homozygous, states 3, 4 and 5 are very similar and states 0 and 3 cannot be differentiated in case of uniparental disomy. (b) Visual interpretation of the states. (c) Transition matrix. The transition probabilities are the probabilities to move from one state for a SNP to another state for the next SNP. The rest of the matrix is given by the detailed balance equation (Durbin et al., 1998). (d) Visual interpretation of the transition parameters. The figure represents two consecutive SNPs in the sample.

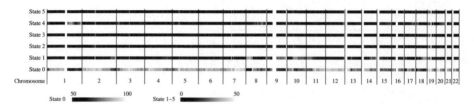

FIG. 3.9: The figure summarizes the 21 tumour samples. The genome is divided into 2 Mb regions and for each sample the frequencies of the different states are counted. Only regions with at least five SNPs are considered. Finally, the frequencies are averaged over the 21 samples. Below is shown the frequency colour code for the different states – note that the percentage of SNPs in state 0 is always >50% and the percentages of the other states always are <50%. State 0: 2 copies (normal unchanged state), 1: heterozygous loss, 2: homozygous loss, 3: uniparental disomy 4: unbalanced amplification, and 5: balanced amplification.

the HMM on all SNPs and then subsequently re-running the HMM on the SNPs that appeared normal in the germline. On average this amounts to approximately 43,000 SNPs per sample, or 78% of the available SNPs. The excluded SNPs (22%) are either not conforming to the model, experimentally unsuccessfull, or in a chromosomal region subject to copy number variation in the germline.

The results are summarized in Fig. 3.9. The genome is divided in 2 Mb regions and for each sample and region the frequency of SNPs in a given state $(0, 1, \ldots, 5)$ is counted. Subsequently, the frequencies of the different states are averaged over the 21 bladder tumour samples. This does not show how the states vary within a single sample, but how the states vary in the tumour population and what the predominant states are.

From Fig. 3.9 it transpires that apart from state 0 (both copies retained), the two most frequent events are loss of a region (LOH) or amplification of a region, often the region extends to an entire chromosome arm. Loss of the p-arm on chromosome 8 is a frequent event in bladder cancer and the majority of the samples have lost the entire arm or part of the arm. Far fewer samples have lost the p-arm of chromosome 17 – the chromosome that harbours the tumour suppressor gene TP53.

Some samples show evidence of uniparental disomy (state 3). On 1q four samples display uniparental disomy and two of these samples are also in state 3 in a region near a putative TSG fumarate hydratase (FH) (according to the OMIM database of disease genes). However, the FH gene itself does not appear to be in the region. Uniparental disomy would be one way to obtain two inactivated copies of a TSG while maintaining the overall integrity of the chromosomal region. Likewise, three samples are in state 3 in a region near the TSG TP53, but again the gene itself is not included. No other TSGs or oncogenes appear to be in regions that show uniparental disomy. Figure 3.10 gives another example

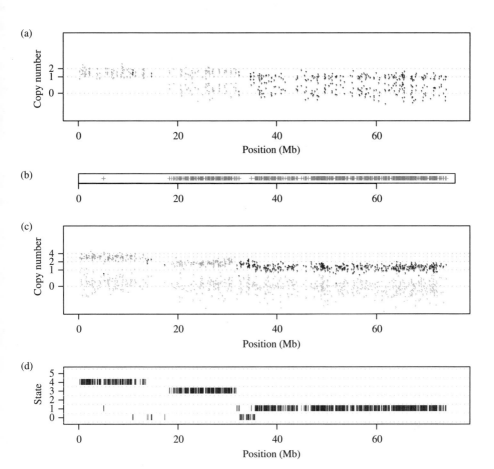

FIG. 3.10: An example of the HMM applied to chromosome 18 in a bladder tumour sample. In this chromosome, we can distinguish uniparental disomy coloured in purple in a region of approximatively 15 Mb and LOH in the rest of the q-arm coloured in blue. In addition, the p-arm has experienced an unbalanced amplification, coloured in orange. (a) For each SNP heterozygous in the germline DNA, the normalized intensities of each allele are plotted. The colours represent the estimated state of the SNP: black for state 0, blue for state 1, green for state 2, purple for state 3, orange for state 4 and red for state 5. (b) Shown is the region of LOH. (c) For each SNP homozygous in the germline DNA, the normalized intensities of each allele are plotted. The absent allele is coloured in grey. (d) Shown is the estimated sequence of hidden states. The colour indicates the posterior probabilities of the states: blue > 0.99, green > 0.95, orange > 0.9 and red < 0.9. See Plate 1.

of uniparental disomy. For the method to be successful an abnormal region needs to extent over several SNPs to be detected.

3.7 Conclusion

We have demonstrated how LOH and allelic copy numbers can be derived statistically with the help of HMMs. A HMM is a very flexible tool that is suitable to model dependent data such as SNP markers where neighbour SNPs are likely to share the same copy number. Unless the signal is very strong small regions in abnormal states are potentially missed because of experimental noise and modelling inaccuracy. As shown in the example above local changes in allelic copy numbers can be difficult to detect unless they extend over a number of SNPs. With the advent of arrays with very high SNP density and better experimental procedures, future methods for allelic copy number determination may improve on this.

References

Andersen, C. L., Wiuf, C., Kruhoffer, M., Korsgaard, M., Laurberg, S., and Orntoft, T. F. (2007). Frequent occurrence of uniparental disomy in colorectal cancer. *Carcinogenesis*, **28**, 38–48.

Bignell, G. R., Huang, J., Greshock, J., Watt, S., Butler, A., West, S., Grigorova, M., Jones, K. W., Wei, W., Stratton, M. R., Futreal, F. A., Weber, B., Shapero, M. H., and Wooster, R. (2004). High-resolution analysis of DNA copy number using oligonucleotide microarrays. *Genome Research*, **14**, 287–295.

Carvalho, B., Bengtsson, H., Speed, T. P, and Irizarry, R. (2007). Exploration, normalization, and genotype calls of high-density oligonucleotide snp array data. *Biostatistics*, **8**, 485–499.

Draghici, S. (2003). *Data Analysis for DNA Microarrays*. Chapman & Hall, New York.

Durbin, R., Eddy, S., Krigh, A., and Mitchison, G. (1998). *Biological Sequence Analysis*. Cambridge University Press, Cambridge.

Ferguson, D. O., Sekiguchi, J. M., Chang, S., Frank, K. M., Gao, Y., DePinho, R. A., and Alt, F. W. (2000). The nonhomologous end-joining pathway of dna repair is required for genomic stability and the suppression of translocations. *Proceedings of the National Academy of Science, USA*, **97**, 6630–6633.

Fridlyand, J., Snijders, A. M., Pinkel, D., Albertson, D. G., and Jain, A. N. (2004). Hidden markov models to approach to the analysis of array cgh data. *Journal of Multivariate Analysis*, **90**, 132–153.

Gaasenbeek, M., Howarth, K., Rowan, A. J., Gorman, P. A., Jones, A., Chaplin, T., Liu, Y., Bicknell, D., Davison, E. J., Fiegler, H., Carter, N. P., Roylance, R. R., and Tomlinson, I. P. (2006). Combined array-comparative genomic hybridization and single-nucleotide polymorphism-loss of heterozygosity analysis reveals complex changes and multiple forms of chromosomal instability in colorectal cancers. *Cancer Research*, **66**, 3471–3479.

Gisselsson, D., Pettersson, L., Hoglund, M., Heidenblad, M., Gorunova, L., Wiegant, J., Mertens, F., Dal Cin, P., Mitelman, F., and Mandahl, N. (2000). Chromosomal breakage-fusion-bridge events cause genetic intratumor heterogeneity. *Proceedings of the National Academy of Science, USA*, **97**, 5357–5362.

Hanahan, D. and Weinberg, R. A. (2000). The hallmarks of cancer. *Cell*, **7**, 57–70.

Huang, J., Wei, W., Chen, J., Zhang, J., Liu, G., Di, X., Mei, R., Ishikawa, S., Aburatani, H., Jones, K. W., and Shapero, M. H. (2006). Carat: a novel method for allelic detection of dna copy number changes using high density oligonucleotide arrays. *BMC Bioinformatics*, **7**, 83.

Ishikawa, S., Komura, D., Tsuji, S., Nishimura, K., Yamamoto, S., Panda, B., Huang, J., Fukayama, M., Jones, K. W., and Aburatani, H. (2006). Carat: a novel method for allelic detection of dna copy number changes using high density oligonucleotide arrays. *BMC Bioinformatics*, **7**, 83.

Jenner, M. W., Leone, P. E., Walker, B. A., Ross, F. M., Johnson, D. C., Gonzalez, D., Chiecchio, L., Dachs Cabanas, E., Dagrada, G. P., Nightingale, M., Protheroe, R. K., Stockley, D., Else, M., Dickens, N. J., Cross, N. C., Davies, F. E., and Morgan, G. J. (2007). Gene mapping and expression analysis of 16q loss of heterozygosity identifies wwox and cyld as being important in determining clinical outcome in multiple myeloma. *Blood*, **110**, 3291–3300.

Kaloshi, G., Benouaich-Amiel, A., Diakite, F., Taillibert, S., Lejeune, J., Laigle-Donadey, F., Renard, M. A, Iraqi, W., Idbaih, A., Paris, S., Capelle, L., Duffau, H., Cornu, P., Simon, J. M, Mokhtari, K., Polivka, M., Omuro, A., Carpentier, A., Sanson, M., Delattre, J. Y, and Hoang-Xuan, K. (2007). Temozolomide for low-grade gliomas: predictive impact of 1p/19q loss on response and outcome. *Neurology*, **68**, 1831–1836.

Knudson, A. (1971). Mutation and cancer: statistical study of retinoblastoma. *Proceedings of the National Academy of Science, USA*, **68**, 820–823.

Koed, K., Wiuf, C., Christensen, L. L., Wikman, F. P., Zieger, K., Moller, K., von der Maase, H., and Orntoft, T. F. (2005). High-density single nucleotide polymorphism array defines novel stage and location-dependent allelic imbalances in human bladder tumors. *Cancer Res*, **65**, 34–45.

LaFramboise, T., Weir, B. A., Zhao, X., Beroukhim, R., Li, C., Harrington, D., Sellers, W. R., and Meyerson, M. (2005). Allele-specific amplification in cancer revealed by snp array analysis. *PLoS Comput Biol*, **1**, e65.

Lamy, P., Andersen, C. L., Wikman, F. P., and Wiuf, C. (2006). Genotyping and annotation of affymetrix snp arrays. *Nucleic Acids Res*, **34**, e100.

Lamy, P., Andersen, C. L, Dyrskjot, L., Torring, N., and Wiuf, C. (2007). A hidden markov model to estimate population mixture and allelic copy-numbers in cancers using affymetrix snp arrays. *BMC Bioinformatics*, **8**, 434.

Lin, M., Wei, L. J., Sellers, W. R., Lieberfarb, M., Wong, W. H., and Li, C. (2004). dchipsnp: significance curve and clustering of snp-array-based loss-of-heterozygosity data. *Bioinformatics*, **20**, 1233–1240.

Li, C. and Wong, W. H. (2001). Model-based analysis of oligonucleotide arrays: expression index computation and outlier detection. *Proceedings of the National Academy of Science, USA*, **98**, 31–36.

Merlo, L. M, Pepper, J. W., Reid, B. J, and Maley, C. C (2006). Cancer as an evolutionary and ecological process. *Nature Reviews Cancer*, **6**, 924–935.

Nannya, Y., Sanada, M., Nakazaki, K., Hosoya, N., Wang, L., Hangaishi, A., Kurokawa, M., Chiba, S., Bailey, D. K., Kennedy, G. C., and Ogawa, S. (2005). A robust algorithm for copy number detection using high-density oligonucleotide single nucleotide polymorphism genotyping arrays. *Cancer Res*, **65**, 6071–6079.

Newton, M. A and Lee, Y. (2000). Inferring the location and effect of tumor suppressor genes by instability-selection modeling of allelic-loss data. *Biometrics*, **56**, 1088–1097.

Rabbee, N. and Speed, T. P. (2006). A genotype calling algorithm for affymetrix snp arrays. *Bioinformatics*, **22**, 7–12.

Redon, R., Ishikawa, S., Fitch, K. R., Feuk, L., Perry, G. H., Andrews, T. D., Fiegler, H., Shapero, M. H., Carson, A. R, Chen, W., Cho, E. K., Dallaire, S., Freeman, J. L., Gonzalez, J. R., Gratacos, M., Huang, J., Kalaitzopoulos, D., Komura, D., MacDonald, J. R., Marshall, C. R., Mei, R., Montgomery, L., Nishimura, K., Okamura, K., Shen, F., Somerville, M. J., Tchinda, J., A.Valsesia, Woodwark, C., Yang, F., Zhang, J., Zerjal, T., Zhang, J., Armengol, L., Conrad, D. F., Estivill, X., Tyler-Smith, C., Carter, N. P., Aburatani, H., Lee, C., Jones, K. W., Scherer, S. W., and Hurles, M. E. (2006). Global variation in copy number in the human genome. *Nature*, **444**, 444–454.

Sarli, L., Bottarelli, L., Bader, G., Iusco, D., Pizzi, S., Costi, R., D'Adda, T., Bertolani, M., Roncoroni, L., and Bordi, C. (2004). Association between recurrence of sporadic colorectal cancer, high level of microsatellite instability, and loss of heterozygosity at chromosome 18q. *Dis Colon Rectum*, **47**, 1467–1482.

Speed, T. (ed.) (2003). *Statistical Analysis of Gene Expression Microarray Data*. Chapman & Hall, New York.

Thiagalingam, S., Laken, S., Willson, J. K, Markowitz, S. D, Kinzler, K. W, Vogelstein, B., and Lengauer, C. (2001). Mechanisms underlying losses of heterozygosity in human colorectal cancers. *Proceedings of the National Academy of Science, USA*, **98**, 2698–2702.

Vogelstein, B. and Kinzler, K. W (2004). Cancer genes and the pathways they control. *Nature Medicine*, **10**, 789–799.

Watanabe, T., Wu, T. T, Catalano, P. J, Ueki, T., Satriano, R., Haller, D. G, Benson, A. B 3rd, and Hamilton, S. R (2001). Molecular predictors of survival after adjuvant chemotherapy for colon cancer. *New England Journal of Medicine*, **344**, 1196–1206.

Weinberg, R. A (2007). *The Biology of Cancer*. Garland Science, New York.

White, S. J., Vissers, L. E. L. M., Geurts van Kessel, A., de Menezes, R. X, Kalay, E., Lehesjoki, A. E., Giordano, P. C., van de Vosse, E., Breuning, M. H., Brunner, H. G., den Dunnen, J. T., and Veltman, J. A. (2007). Variation of cnv distribution in five different ethnic populations. *Cytogenet Genome Res*, **118**, 19–30.

Zieger, K., Dyrskjot, L., Wiuf, C., Jensen, J. L., Andersen, C. L., Jensen, K. M., and Orntoft, T. F. (2005). Role of activating fibroblast growth factor receptor 3 mutations in the development of bladder tumors. *Clin Cancer Res*, **11**, 7709–7719.

4

BIOINFORMATICS OF GENE EXPRESSION AND COPY NUMBER DATA INTEGRATION

Outi Monni and Sampsa Hautaniemi

4.1 Introduction

Transcription is a process by which inheritable information encoded in our DNA is transformed into messenger RNA (mRNA). mRNA is further translated into a functional gene product (protein). Gene expression in a cell can be studied by measuring relative quantities of mRNA molecules. mRNA constitutes only 1–2% of total RNA. Total RNA also contains transfer RNA (tRNA) and ribosomal RNA (rRNA) that have a role in protein translation as well as a number of different small RNAs, such as siRNAs and miRNAs that have a role in gene regulation. In each cell type, only a set of genes (about 30–50% of the genes in the genome) are expressed at any given time. Each tissue has its specific gene expression profile. Gene expression is influenced by a number of cellular and external factors. For example, some of the genes are expressed only in certain developmental stage or in response to specific external stimuli.

As compared to the RNA, DNA is much more stable. In normal situation, each individual has 46 chromosomes including 22 pairs of autosomes and two sex chromosomes XX (female) or XY (male). In cancers, normal cellular growth control is disturbed, which causes problems in cell division. This may give rise to either losses (deletions) or gains (amplifications) of chromosome numbers or chromosomal regions. These additions or losses of genetic material are called copy number changes or alterations. The gains typically contain genes that are important for example in promotion of the cell growth or inhibition of apoptosis, whereas lost regions may contain genes that are important for example in DNA damage signalling, promotion of apoptosis or control of the cell cycle.

Both the genetic information encoded in our DNA and gene expression (mRNA) are altered in cancer. When the copy number or gene expression levels are compared with the normal situation, it is possible to receive information on the genes that are likely to have importance in cancer development.

It is well-known that gene copy number alterations play an important role in cancer development and progression (Knuutila et al., 1999). The frequency of copy number alterations varies between different cancers, but they are particularly common in solid tumours, such as in cancers of breast, prostate, lung, gastric, ovarian, pancreas and head and neck (Knuutila et al., 1999). In different tumours, the number, size and magnitude of copy number alterations vary extensively and that is likely to reflect the differences of individual tumours to escape from normal protective cellular environment (Fridlyand et al., 2006).

Gene amplification is an important mechanism for the cancer cells to increase the expression of cellular proto-oncogenes. Similarly, gene deletions and simultaneous decrease in gene expression may turn off critical tumour suppressor genes that are mutated in their other allele (Knudson, 2001).

The impact of gene copy number on gene expression varies between different cancers. For example, recent studies have shown that up to 40–50% of the highly amplified genes are also over-expressed in cancer (Pollack et al., 1999; Hyman et al., 2002; Järvinen et al., 2006). The impact of deletion on underexpression is less clear, which is partly due to the fact that small deletions and following underexpression is technically more challenging to identify. In general, it has been demonstrated that 10–15% of all gene expression changes are directly associated with gene copy number changes (Pollack et al., 2002; Hyman et al., 2002; Järvinen et al., 2006). The identification of the genes that are either amplified and overexpressed or deleted and underexpressed may reveal alterations critical to tumour pathogenesis.

A number of methods have been developed to measure copy number and gene expression levels on a genome-wide basis in cancer. In this chapter, we will first briefly review methods that can be used in global detection of copy number and gene expression levels, and then concentrate on discussing how microarrays can be used to integrate the data from both the copy number and gene expression measurements.

4.2 Methods

4.2.1 Methods to study copy number levels

Gene copy number levels can be studied on a genome-wide basis by several different methods. Traditionally, chromosomal alterations have been studied by conventional G-banding technique, also called karyotyping, where chromosomes are stained with Giemsa staining at the metaphase phase of the cell division (mitosis). This staining produces a G-banding called a staining pattern by which chromosomes can be identified. The technique has several limitations. For example, cancer cells need to be cultured *in vitro*, which is challenging especially for solid tumours. Additionally, karyotypes of tumours are often very chaotic with a number of numerical and structural chromosomal alterations, which makes the identification of the chromosomal alterations very challenging. G-banding is neither very sensitive in detecting small copy number alterations and in general, less than 10–20 Mb alterations remain undetected.

In the early 1990s, the technique called comparative genomic hybridization (CGH) was developed for mapping the copy number alterations in cancer cells for normal metaphase chromosomes (Kallioniemi et al., 1992). This technology has revolutionizing cancer research, since it allows the study of those tumour types that were difficult to cultivate *in vitro*. This technique is based on the comparison of differentially labelled (for example red and green fluorescence dyes) test and reference DNAs that are simultaneously hybridized on normal chromosomes. The labelled sequences find their complementary sequences on the chromosomes and bind to these sequences in a competitive manner. If the test sample is labelled with red fluorescence colour, those sequences that are amplified in test sample (for example in cancer specimen), show increased red fluorescence ratio. Losses of sequences in the test sample are detected as increased green colour. The resolution of this technique is better than with chromosomal karyotyping, but it is still not very sensitive for detecting small copy number alterations, especially small deletions (resolution 2–10 Mb). However, the technique is very useful in detection of large unbalanced chromosomal alterations and high-level amplifications.

In addition to G-banding and chromosomal CGH, other methods can be applied to study copy number alterations. For example, spectral karyotyping, which was developed after the discovery of fluorescence *in situ* hybridization (FISH) and CGH, is based on the fluorescence staining of each chromosome or chromosome arm with different fluorochromes (Schrock et al., 1996). This technique allows the detection of extra or missing copies of chromosomal material, but does not give exact information about the genes involved in the altered regions.

4.2.2 Methods to study gene expression

Different methods can be applied to study gene expression levels on a genome-wide manner. These methods include for example serial analysis of gene expression (SAGE), differential display, and gene expression microarrays, the latter of which will be described later in more detail in this chapter.

SAGE relies on the sequencing of short cDNA sequences without requirement of any *a priori* knowledge of the genes to be studied (Velculescu et al., 1995). SAGE is practically based on sequencing of every transcript in a cell or tissue providing qualitative and quantitative data of gene expression levels. SAGE is based on detection of 9 to 10 base pair nucleotide sequence tags that uniquely identify a transcript. Concatenation of these short sequence tags allows the efficient analysis of transcripts in a serial manner by sequencing of multiple tags within a single clone. The advantage of the method is that it produces quantitative data, but the sequencing of the transcripts is very labour-intensive.

Differential display is a technique that was invented in 1992 to allow the detection of gene expression alterations between two different biological conditions, typically diseased and normal tissue (Liang and Pardee, 1992). Like SAGE, differential display provides quantitative data of the gene expression measurements across the whole genome. In this method, reverse transcription and polymerase chain reaction are first applied to separate and clone individual messenger RNAs (mRNAs) in two different samples using a poly-dT primer that anneals to the 3′ end of mRNAs and a random primer that is short and arbitrary in sequence and anneals to different positions in mRNA transcript relative to the first primer. The identified mRNA sequences defined by these primer pairs are then run on a DNA sequencing gel. Different bands in the gel can then be isolated, cloned and sequenced to identify transcripts that are differentially expressed between two conditions. Like SAGE, the method produces quantitative data, but the analysis of multiple samples can take several weeks.

4.2.3 *Microarrays in detection of copy number and gene expression levels*

DNA microarrays can be used to study both the gene expression levels and copy number alterations. The technique provides a fast and easy way to identify expression or copy number levels of all the genes in a genome in one laboratory experiment. Microarrays were initially developed to study differentially expressed genes (Schena et al., 1995; Lockhart et al., 1996), but the technique can also be applied to study relative quantities of practically any biomolecule in a cell. Gene expression microarrays consist typically of 200–10,000 base pair PCR products or 25–80 long oligonucleotide sequences arrayed or *in situ* synthesized on a solid support, such as glass. One transcript can be represented by long oligos or a number of short oligonucleotide probes, the intensity of which is then combined when the array is analysed. Transcripts can also be represented by pairs of perfect and mismatch oligos. The intensity of a specific signal can then be compared to an unspecific signal which further improves the accuracy of the analysis. Microarrays can be constructed by spotting DNA on a microscope slide using particular arrayers or alternatively, microarrays can be obtained from commercial vendors. After the technology was first developed, a number of academic groups constructed their own microarrays using large cDNA clone libraries. However, due to the problems in well-to-well contamination when handling these libraries in 96- or 384-well format, currently nearly all commercial manufacturers synthesize or spot 25-80 base oligonucleotides on a solid support. Gene expression microarrays have applications in nearly all fields of biomedical research. The technology has been mostly applied in cancer research, including disease classification, drug discovery, pharmacogenomics, toxicity profiling of new drugs and also in diagnostics.

When DNA microarrays are applied to study copy number alterations, the technique is called array-CGH (aCGH) or CGH microarray because it is based on the same principle as chromosomal CGH. In this technique however, small DNA fragments are used as targets instead of metaphase chromosomes. CGH microarrays are typically constructed from large genomic BAC clones (100–300kb in size), cDNAs or oligonucleotides (Solinas-Toldo et al., 1997; Pinkel et al., 1998; Pollack et al., 1999). The advantage of using large genomic clones as targets on the array is better sensitivity, but oligo arrays allow better resolution and specificity due to the smaller size of the probe on the array. Therefore, oligonucleotide arrays can be applied to study small homozygous deletions or intragenic copy number variations consisting of only a part of the gene. The aCGH technology has a number of different applications. It has been mostly used in basic research to study gene copy number alterations in diseases like cancer and mental retardation, but currently there are also examples utilizing array-CGH in comparative genomics and diagnostics.

4.3 Microarray experiment

The principle of the gene expression microarray technique is to compare the relative abundance of expressed sequences between different samples. In a microarray experiment, one can study for example the differential expression across a series of tumour samples or compare gene expression levels between treated and non-treated samples. Gene expression microarrays can either be carried out as a two-colour or one-colour experiment. In a two-colour experiment, test and reference RNAs extracted from two samples are labelled with two different fluorescent colours (typically Cy3 and Cy5) and hybridized simultaneously on a microscope slide. This experiment provides ratio data between the test and reference sample. Alternatively, only one sample can be labelled and hybridized on a microarray which produces intensity data instead of ratios.

Array-CGH is normally carried out as a two-colour experiment where the DNA sample extracted from the studied sample is hybridized against normal DNA. To avoid false positive results, reference DNA should be a pool of normal DNAs extracted from different individuals due to the copy number variation that has recently been found to occur also in normal population (Iafrate et al., 2004; Sebat et al., 2004). Test and reference DNAs are typically labelled with Cy3 and Cy5 fluorescent labels.

After the hybridization, microarrays are scanned with a microarray scanner that produces a 16-bit image file. Various image processing software can then be used to transform the image data into numerical format. These image analysis software packages are also often used in initial microarray analysis, especially in background correction and normalization of the data. There is a large number of different image processing software packages available, but typically each microarray platform has its own image analysis software recommended by the manufacturer.

After scanning of the microarray slide that produces a 16-bit image, each gene on the array is summarized by two intensity values that are typically the mean or median of all pixel intensity values on the spot. These values belong to $[0, \ldots, 65535]$. Even though intensity values are often used in microarray data quality control, they are rarely used in actual analysis (except when the microarray format is single-colour). In two-colour experiments the two intensity estimates are divided to form ratios. Formally, the raw ratio for the ith gene on the array is:

$$r_i = \frac{I_i^t}{I_i^r}, \qquad (4.1)$$

where I_i^t is the test signal intensity (Cy3 labelled sample), and I_i^r the reference signal intensity (Cy5 labeled sample). Practically, test and reference samples can be labelled using either Cy3 or Cy5, so prior analysis is crucial to check whether Cy3 is test or reference. After a microarray experiment, the obtained raw ratios are preprocessed to be used in data analysis.

If one is interested in identification of genes where change in gene expression is associated with copy number alteration, CGH and gene expression microarray data can be integrated. In Fig. 4.1 we show an example where DNAs and RNAs

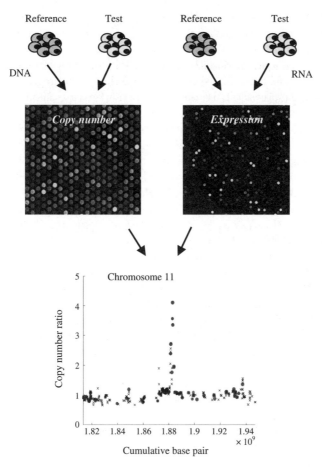

FIG. 4.1: To study gene expression alterations that are associated with DNA copy number alterations, DNA and RNA can be extracted from the same sample and hybridized on both the gene expression and CGH microarrays. An example of a microarray experiment, where the data has been integrated using an expression annotated copy number (ECN) tool for chromosome 11 is shown. This sample shows high-level amplication of 11q13. See Plate 2.

isolated from an identical tissue sample are hybridized on a gene expression and CGH microarrays. The data can then be visualized by colour-coded copy number plots, where the X-axis shows the genomic position of the probes on an array and the Y-axis shows the copy number ratio. Red colour indicates over-expression in which the gene belongs to the upper 7th percentile of the gene expression ratios in the analysed sample (Fig. 4.1).

Typically, one microarray experiment consists of dozens of samples and since one microarray slide often contains thousands of genes, one microarray produces enormous amounts of data. Therefore, bioinformatics has a central role in a microarray experiment. Various commercial and custom-developed tools have been developed to further analyse and visualize the microarray data. These tools are discussed in more detail in the next section of this chapter in regard to integration of copy number and gene expression data.

A number of studies integrating microarray-based copy number and gene expression data have been published aiming at identification of genes whose expression changes are associated with copy number alterations. In a study by Wolf and co-workers, copy number and gene expression alterations were integrated in four prostate cancer cell lines to map target genes for genetic rearrangements and to study the impact of copy number changes on gene expression (Wolf et al., 2004). In this study, copy number and gene expression analysis was performed on 16K cDNA microarrays including 11,600 cDNA clones mapping across the genome as well as 4700 cDNA clones mapping to common cancer amplicons. These regions included 2p23–p25, 5p, 8q, 10q21–q24, 11q12–q14, 12q13–q15, 17q11.2–q23, 20q, and Xcen–q13. The copy number data were also compared to the data obtained from chromosomal CGH and in this study, 92% of the amplifications and 82% of the deletions identified by chromosomal CGH could be detected by array-based CGH. Additionally, a number of other regions were identified that could not be identified using chromosomal CGH. Altogether, 10.6% of the amplified genes showed an increased gene expression ratio and 6.9% of the genes with normal copy number ratio were up-regulated. On average, gene amplification led to a 2.8-fold increase in over-expressed genes across the studied samples. Similarly, gene deletions led to a 1.8-fold increase in under-expressed genes as compared to genes with normal copy number, demonstrating that copy number alterations (gains and losses) have significant impact on gene expression.

In another study by Järvinen and co-workers (Järvinen et al., 2006), an integrated high-resolution microarray analysis of gene copy number and expression was performed for 20 laryngeal cancer cell lines and primary tumours to identify genetic alterations that would play a key role in disease pathogenesis and pinpoint genes whose expression is impacted by gene copy number alterations. Integration of copy number data from array-based comparative genomic hybridization with gene expression information from oligonucleotide microarrays was performed using custom-developed CGH-Plotter (Autio et al., 2003), which is described in detail later in this chapter. This study showed that copy number alterations and especially high-level amplifications had a clear impact on gene expression. Out of the genes that were in the highest copy number class (> 2), 39% showed over-expression in the cell lines and 18% in the primary tumours. The impact of deletions on the reduced expression was less clear with 14% of genes being under-expressed with copy number ratio of 0.7. Across the genome, over-expression of 739 genes was attributed to gene amplification events in cell lines, with 325 genes showing this association in primary tumours. Integrating the copy number and gene expression data also facilitated the identification of putative targets for copy number alterations. For example, 11q13 amplification is one of the most common highly amplified regions in head and neck cancer and *CCND1* is often considered as a target gene for this region. In a study by Järvinen and colleagues, however, *CCND1* was identified to be often amplified, but not over-expressed in head and neck cancers. Instead, genes called *FADD* and *PPFIA1* were most highly amplified and over-expressed in this region and the over-expression also correlated with increased protein level. Another highly amplified region in head and neck cancer cell lines was at 12q14–21 which contains a well-known oncogene, *MDM2*, that is a regulator of p53 and is often amplified and over-expressed in epithelial cancers. In addition to *MDM2*, a number of other genes in this region were identified as amplified and over-expressed demonstrating that further functional studies are required to determine the target genes for this alteration (Fig. 4.2). The analysis of gene ontology and pathway distributions further pinpointed biological processes and pathways that are impacted due to copy number events. This study highlighted genes that may be critically important to laryngeal cancer progression and suggested potential targets for therapeutic intervention.

To identify which biological processes or pathways are activated due to copy number events, a number of academic and commercial software packages are available to study which Gene Ontology classes or pathways are enriched in a studied data set, as discussed in more detail later in this chapter. For example, a recent study by Myllykangas and co-workers demonstrated an association between over-expression and copy number gain for 657 genes, whereas 95 genes showed an association between under-expression and copy number loss (Myllykangas et al., 2008). When these data were imported into the GeneGO MetaCore pathway software, a number of pathways were shown to be activated by gene amplification. For example, biological pathways involved in signal transduction, translation and ErbB-family signalling were enriched in the integrated data demonstrating that a number of pathways involved in critical cellular processes are activated due to copy number gains.

Integration of gene copy number and gene expression data has proven to be useful in identification of genes that might be targets for copy number alterations as well as putative targets for therapeutic interventions. A classical example of such a drug target is *HER2* (also known as *ERBB2*), which is amplified and over-expressed in 10–30% of breast cancers and patients with this alteration have particularly aggressive disease. Patients with *HER2* amplification and over-expression are treated with Herceptin antibody-based therapy that blocks dimerization of ERBB2 with other ErbB-family members and prevents it from transmitting growth signals to the cell. Due to the recent development of many novel genome-wide technologies, it is likely that similar examples of therapies targeting specific genetic alteration will appear also in the near future.

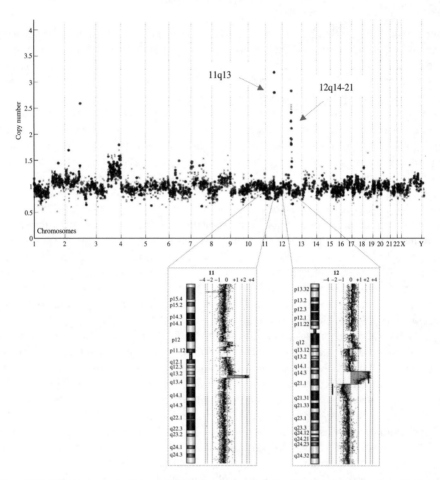

FIG. 4.2: Gene-expression annotated copy number plot for head and neck squamous cell carcinoma cell line. All the cDNA clones on array-CGH are arranged on the X-axis according to their base-pair position in the genome. The Y-axis shows the copy number ratio for each clone. If the ratio exceeds 1.3, the gene is regarded as amplified and if it is below 0.7, the gene is regarded as deleted. The color-coding indicates the gene expression ratio of each gene on a microarray. Red indicates over-expression, whereas green indicates under-expression. This figure illustrates that most of the genes in highly amplified regions show increased gene expression ratio. Below the expression-annotated copy number plot are shown the corresponding high-resolution copy number profiles for two highly amplified regions, 11q13 and 12q14-21, using oligonucleotide array that consists of 185,000 oligonucleotides on a single array. These views show that a number of genes are located in highly amplified regions. See Plate 3.

4.4 Analysis and integration of gene expression and copy number data

A major objective for studies integrating high-throughput gene expression and copy number data is to identify genes that are either amplified and over-expressed or deleted and under-expressed since these can be attributed to cancer initiation and progression.

In general, identification of amplified and over-expressed genes is easier than that of deleted and under-expressed genes. The reason is that signal intensity for an over-expressed or amplified gene can be very high, such as 2^{16} for 16-bit images, whereas for down-regulated or deleted genes the signal can be 0. That is, for over-expressed or amplified genes the signal strength can be very high compared to the noise level, and is relatively straightforward to detect. However, the signal-to-noise ratio for a down-regulated or deleted gene can be low, and creates challenges to separate the signal from the noise. As an exact model for noise in microarray experiments is still an open problem, various signal processing methods to tackle the noise issue may need to be applied when identifying under-expressed or deleted genes.

4.4.1 *Preprocessing*

All microarray data should be carefully preprocessed before analysis. In this section, we describe briefly standard preprocessing principles and methods. A more detailed description of the methods is given in the microarray literature, such as in Draghici (2003).

The exact preprocessing steps depend on the microarray platform and the experimental design. For example, two-colour arrays require correction for dye-bias between the two channels (Cy3 and Cy5) which is due to different chemical properties of the two dyes (called dye-bias correction) and different dye emission efficiencies and scanner laser voltage settings. The three major steps that are common for all array platforms are: *quality control, within-slide normalization* and *between-slides normalization*.

4.4.1.1 *Two-colour microarray experimental design*
In a two-colour microarray experiment one of the most important steps is to choose a reference sample for the microarray experiment. One option is to use a universal reference, such as a pool of different cancer cell lines. The idea of using a pool of cancer cell lines as a reference sample is to have as many genes expressed as possible, so measurement points can be theoretically obtained from a maximum number of features per array. As each test sample is compared to the same reference sample, both the experimental design and the data preprocessing are relatively straightforward.

From a statistical experimental design point of view the reference design may not be as effective as more complicated designs, such as loop design and dye-swap design (Kerr and Churchill, 2001). The more complex designs, however, often require twice as many experiments as compared to the reference design. To date, all studies integrating gene expression and copy number data from two-colour arrays have used a reference design and therefore we will only discuss the reference design. A discussion of preprocessing data emerging from other designs is given elsewhere (Altman and Hua, 2006).

4.4.1.2 *Quality control* A typical microarray experiment results in more than one million data points. If only 0.1% of the data is erroneous, there will still be over 1000 spurious values. As currently the error rates for microarray experiments are much higher than 0.1%, the microarray data should always be quality controlled before proceeding to further analyses. Quality control is particularly important for studies integrating copy number and gene expression data due to biological reasons. The range of intensities in copy number data is much lower than with gene expression values. More than a 10-fold relative increase in gene expression can often be identified between two conditions, whereas such a high increase in relative copy number is uncommon even in tumour samples.

The major objective for quality control is to identify features (or spots) that are considered to be unreliable. Possible sources for unreliable spots are dust, dye bursts, bleeding, or problems in microarray printing. Thus, quality control is an important step to be employed to the scanned images.

The simplest quality control method is to use thresholds for signal intensity and spot size. For example, a spot is flagged as unreliable if signal intensity in both channels is below 100 fluorescent units, or the size of the spot is under 50 pixels (Hyman *et al.*, 2002). These cut-offs depend on the microarray platform and hybridization protocol. More sophisticated methods to automatically detect bad quality spots from microarray images have been reported, for instance, by Hautaniemi *et al.* (2003) and Zhang *et al.* (2004).

After the quality control step, the microarray data can be represented as a matrix. Let the gene expression data matrix be $\mathbf{E}_q \in \mathbb{R}^{m \times M}$ and the copy number data matrix be $\mathbf{C}_q \in \mathbb{R}^{n \times N}$, where the subscript q denotes quality controlled, m and n the numbers of genes in the gene expression and copy number experiments, respectively; and M and N the number of samples in the gene expression and copy number experiments, respectively.

4.4.1.3 *Within-slide normalization* Within-slide normalization methods aim to ensure that the values in each column in the quality controlled data matrices $\mathbf{E}_q, \mathbf{C}_q$ are comparable. The major sources for variation of the values in a microarray experiment include the following: Variation of the amount of DNA in the spots on a microarray (in cDNA microarrays), systematic variation in printing pin groups (print-tip bias), and unequal background intensity of the scanned microarray.

In two-colour microarray experiments, the signal intensity from the test sample is divided by the intensity of the control sample and the downstream analyses are carried out using logarithmically transformed ratios (log-ratios). Formally, the within-slide normalized ratio for the ith gene on a microarray is obtained with the equation:

$$r_i = \frac{I_i^t}{\phi \cdot I_i^r}, \qquad (4.2)$$

where I_i^t and I_i^r are again the test and reference signal intensities, respectively, and ϕ is a normalization factor that is to be estimated by a within-slide normalization method.

Various sources of noise can severely twist the ratio distribution. The basic assumption behind normalization methods is that the expected ratio distribution for microarray data (after taking logarithm) is symmetric with zero mean. The normalization can be performed for example using within-slide normalization with housekeeping genes that are assumed to be constantly expressed in all of the cells. Therefore, the housekeeping normalization method would use the housekeeping gene values to correct all the other values on the microarray (Chen et al., 1997).

Since the expression of housekeeping genes may vary depending on different tissues, a common approach to perform within-slide normalization is to apply the local weighted scatterplot smoother (LOWESS) method to the overall intensity, $A_i = \log_2(\sqrt{I_i^t \cdot I_i^r})$, vs. the logarithm of the ratio, $M_i = \log_2(I_i^t/I_i^r)$, scatterplot (Yang et al., 2001). The (A,M)-scatterplot may reveal artefacts not visible when plotting signal intensities for red and green channels against each other. The LOWESS method consists of four parameters, from which the fraction of data points used in local regression (f) is the most influential. The parameter $f \in [0,1]$, and if f is small the correction is dramatic, whereas a large f produces a small correction. An optimization method to systematically assess the f value is introduced by Berger et al. (2004).

4.4.1.4 *Between-slides normalization* Between-slides normalization is performed after within-slide normalization to ensure that the values across different experiments are comparable. Possible sources causing variation between the microarray experiments include biological and technical variation. In some cases, there can also be variation between microarray slides (batch variation).

The between-slides normalization methods are dependent on the purpose of the study. In studies integrating gene expression and copy number values, it is often enough that the ratios are log-transformed, and minimum, maximum and mean log ratios are in the same range across different experiments. Usually gene expression data and copy number data are normalized separately. The input for the within-slide and between-slides normalization are $\mathbf{E}_q, \mathbf{C}_q$. After normalization, we denote the ratio matrices that are quality controlled, within-slide and between-slide normalized as $\mathbf{E} \in \mathbb{R}^{n \times N}, \mathbf{C} \in \mathbb{R}^{m \times M}$. The matrices $\mathbf{E}$ and $\mathbf{C}$ are used in downstream analyses and may contain missing values.

4.4.2 Identifying amplified and deleted regions from array-CGH data

A fundamental question in the analysis of high-throughput CGH data is to identify regions that are amplified or deleted. This question, however, is non-trivial to solve mainly due to the following reasons. Firstly, highly amplified or deleted single probes are of lesser importance as compared to several modest amplified or deleted probes in the same chromosomal region, rendering methods that test directly single probes inefficient. Secondly, size and amplitude of amplified/deleted regions vary from cancer to cancer. For example, in some cases, amplified regions can be very narrow and amplification may be followed by a deletion; whereas in some other cases, the aberrant regions may be very large, comprising whole chromosome arms. Thirdly, cancers are heterogeneous and often only a subset of samples shares an amplification or deletion. Therefore, simply taking a mean or median of the CGH data across the samples may hide regions that are rare but potentially clinically important for a subset of samples.

There exists a plethora of computational methods to identify deleted or amplified regions in different conditions ranging from fairly straightforward mean filtering (Pollock, 2002) to mathematically more elaborated methods such as dynamic programming and hidden Markov models (Autio et al., 2003; Fridlyand et al., 2004). Notwithstanding the method that has been used to identify amplified and deleted regions, in studies where array-CGH and gene expression data are to be integrated, CGH data are often transformed to nominal variable type (class labels), such as '-1' for deletion, '0' for baseline (no-change) and '1' for amplification. This dimension reduction greatly facilitates the integration of array-CGH and gene expression data. In the data mining literature this kind of dimension reduction is known as segmentation.

Due to the large number of methods to analyse array-CGH data, Lai and colleagues conducted a comparison study of 11 different CGH data analysis algorithms (Lai et al., 2005). They used receiver order characteristic (ROC) analysis to estimate the true positive rate against false positive rate. The overall conclusion is that segmentation based algorithms (Olshen et al., 2004; Picard et al., 2005) perform consistently well. Recently, Lai and colleagues developed a web-based aCGH data analysis package that allows method developers to both test the existing tools and develop novel methods for aCGH data analysis (Lai et al., 2008).

Taken together, the array-CGH data analysis step results in a segmented CGH data matrix $\mathbf{C}_s \in \{-1, 0, 1\}^{n \times N}$. An example of CGH data and CGH-Plotter analysis is shown in Fig. 4.3 for chromosome 1 in prostate cancer cell line PC3. The figure shows three narrow but clear amplifications and large deletion between two amplifications.

4.4.3 *Statistical approach to integrate gene expression and array-CGH data*

In a typical study, where gene expression and CGH data are integrated, the goal is to identify genes whose expression alteration is associated with the gene copy number change. Therefore, standard statistical data analysis tools for identifying differentially expressed genes (DEGs) are of little use in integrative analysis for gene expression and copy number data. A highly expressed gene with high-fold

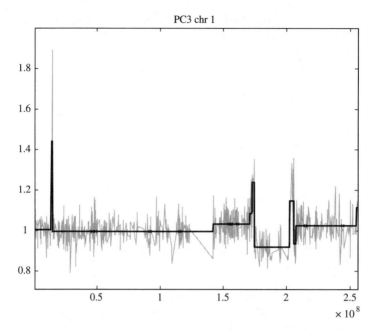

FIG. 4.3: An example of CGH data (grey lines) analysis for chromosome 1 in prostate cancer cell line PC3. The x-axis denotes cumulative base-pairs and the y-axis normalized ratios. The thick solid line is a result from CGH-Plotter analysis (Autio *et al.*, 2003) and crosses denote missing values. The figure illustrates three narrow amplified regions and large deletion between two amplicons in 1.7×10^8–2×10^8 base-pairs.

change or statistical significance for differential expression without amplification in CGH data should not make it to the top list after the integration analysis.

The simplest approach to identify amplified and over-expressed or deleted and down-regulated genes is to correlate CGH data directly to the gene expression data. In such approaches a sliding window over CGH and gene expression data can be used and correlations between the values inside this window are calculated. Chromosomal regions and genes that show high correlation can then be examined in a more detailed fashion. Cancers are heterogeneous and it is not assumed that a gene would be over-expressed and amplified across all samples. Thus, correlation based analyses may not detect genes that share high correlation only in a small subset of samples. Genes being altered only in a subset of samples may still be biologically relevant.

The first systematic approach to integrate gene expression and CGH data so that also subsets of samples are taken into account is introduced in (Hyman *et al.*, 2002; Hautaniemi *et al.*, 2004). This approach assumes that the CGH and gene expression levels are measured from the same sample. That is, the ith sample in the normalized gene expression ratio matrix **E** is the same sample as the ith sample in the normalized CGH data ratio matrix **C**. This implies that $N = M$ and if a gene is not measured on a gene expression or CGH microarray, such values are treated as missing values. Analysis to identify amplified and over-expressed genes is run separately from identifying deleted and down-regulated genes.

After preprocessing the gene expression data, the aCGH ratio data are converted to nominal values (class labels) as described in Section 4.4.2. These labels are used to divide the gene expression values into two classes: amplified and not-changed (deleted and not-changed) depending on the labels. Then, a weight value (w) for each gene on the microarray is computed:

$$w = \frac{m_1 - m_0}{\sigma_1 + \sigma_0}, \qquad (4.3)$$

where m_1 is the mean of the gene expressions for amplified samples based on the labels (similarly for deleted samples), m_0 is the mean of the gene expression values belonging to no-change category based on the CGH data, σ_1 is the standard deviation of the gene expression values for amplified samples and σ_0 the standard deviation for no-change expression values. When identifying deleted and under-expressed genes m_1 and σ_1 are replaced by m_{-1} and σ_{-1}. Further details are discussed in Hautaniemi *et al.* (2004).

The weight value (w) is large when amplified (deleted) and gene expression values are clearly distinct from the 'no-change' gene expression values, and variation in both classes is small. Due to the sum of the standard deviations in the denominator, eqn (4.3) may rank high genes with extremely similar expression values across all the samples. As these genes are not of interest, a statistical measure called the α-value is computed for each gene. The α-value tells the probability that the null-hypothesis 'large weight is due to a random event' is erroneously rejected. Statistical computations are done using a permutation test, where the labels are randomly permuted and the weight is computed for the permuted class labels with eqn (4.3). If the randomly permuted weight is greater than or equal to the original weight, then a counter is incremented by one. The counter is divided by the number of permutations. For instance, if 10,000 permutations are run and the randomly permutated weight was 100 times greater than or equal to original weight, the α-value is $100/10000 = 0.01$.

After the permutation test, each gene receives weight and significance values. The genes with the highest weight and the lowest α-value are the most likely candidates to have over-expression (down-regulation) due to amplification (deletion). A schematic of the approach is given in Fig. 4.4.

4.4.3.1 *An application of the statistical approach to integrate gene expression and array-CGH data* The statistical approach to combine CGH data with gene expression values has been applied to the analysis of several cancer types, including neuroblastoma, pancreas, breast, gastric, prostate, and head and neck cancers. The statistical integration of CGH data and gene expression values does

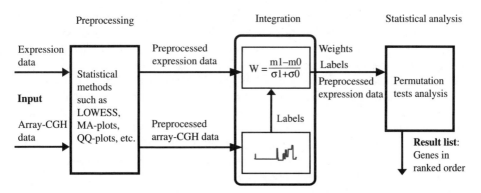

FIG. 4.4: Flow diagram for integration of CGH and gene expression data. First, the data are preprocessed. Second, CGH data are analysed in order to identify amplified, no-change and deleted regions. For each gene the analysis results in class labels indicating whether the gene is amplified, deleted or not changed in a particular sample. The labels are used to divide gene expression data into amplified (deleted) vs. no-change groups. Third, a weight for each gene is computed with eqn (4.3). Fourth, a permutation test is used to compute the α-value that tells the probability that the null-hypothesis 'large weight is due to a random event' is erroneously rejected. The result of the integrative analysis is a list of prioritized genes whose expression changes are likely due to copy number variation. These genes are then annotated with, for instance, pathway and Gene Ontology analysis.

not require non-cancerous reference samples, although if such are available they can be used to form the ratios as described in eqn (4.1). As each weight value is associated with α-value that is computed with a permutation test, the minimum number of samples is five. Further, as the labels for CGH data are permuted, genes that are amplified or deleted in all samples still get α-value of zero regardless of their gene expression values. Thus, an analyst needs to manually check expression levels for genes that are amplified or deleted in all samples. Typically the number of such genes is small (<30 genes). The statistical approach tolerates missing values well as long as the number of samples with non-missing values for genes having both gene expression and copy number measurement is at least five.

Equation (4.3) and associated α-value were applied for integration of CGH data and gene expression values for the first time by Hyman *et al.* (2002). The authors used 14 breast cancer cell lines whose CGH and gene expression levels were measured for 13,000 genes using cDNA two-colour microarrays. The analysis resulted in 270 genes that are both amplified and over-expressed in breast cancer. This gene set includes several genes that have been previously described as breast cancer genes as well as novel candidates, such as the *HOXB7* gene, whose amplification was identified to be clinically associated with poor patient prognosis.

Hyman et al. (2002) used a 5% threshold to determine amplified genes from the CGH data. That is, the highest 5% of the values in **C** are labelled with '1' and the rest with '0'. Note that the objective was to identify amplified and over-expressed genes, so also deleted CGH values are labelled with '0'. Even though the use of such a threshold yielded biologically relevant results, the analysis would probably benefit from a more systematic way to identify amplified genes from CGH data. Thus, a re-analysis of the same 14 breast cancer cell lines was carried out to identify amplified genes using CGH-Plotter (Autio et al., 2003) as described by Hautaniemi et al. (2004). The re-analysis resulted in 92 genes that were both amplified and over-expressed in breast cancer. This set included previously described breast cancer genes and several novel candidate genes, including *HOXB7*. The main reason for the differences between these two resulting gene lists is in the labelling step. In the re-analysis, criteria for a gene to be considered amplified were more stringent that in the original study.

4.4.4 Data reduction model approach to integrate gene expression and array-CGH data

Methods that segment the array-CGH data prior to integrating the CGH data to gene expression levels have resulted in impressive results, but suffer from high dependency on the segmentation step. Segmentation of noisy CGH data is a non-trivial endeavour, and a user needs to adjust several parameters that often determine the performance of the integration analysis. Given the high heterogeneity between, for example, different cancers, array platforms and sample materials, proper tuning of the segmentation parameter is challenging.

CGH data segmentation is often laborious and error prone, so alternative integrative approaches that do not apply segmentation to the CGH data have been suggested. First a systematic approach to integrate gene expression and CGH data without segmentation is the data reduction model approach suggested in Berger et al. (2006). The basic idea behind this approach is to iteratively decompose both gene expression and CGH data using the generalized singular value decomposition (GSVD) relying on singular value decomposition (SVD). SVD is a factorization method in linear algebra and it has been used successfully in numerous applications. For example, in principal component analysis the SVD is generally used as a numerically stable way to compute the principal components.

Assume a preprocessed gene expression matrix $\mathbf{E} = [\mathbf{e}_1, \ldots, \mathbf{e}_M]$. The SVD theorem (Golub and Loan, 1996) states that there exists orthogonal matrices

$$\mathbf{U} = (\mathbf{u}_1, \ldots, \mathbf{u}_m) \in \mathbb{R}^{m \times m}$$

and

$$\mathbf{V} = (\mathbf{v}_1, \ldots, \mathbf{v}_M) \in \mathbb{R}^{M \times M}$$

such that

$$\mathbf{U}^T \mathbf{E} \mathbf{V} = \mathrm{diag}(\sigma_1, \ldots, \sigma_M) \in \mathbb{R}^{m \times M}$$

where $\sigma_1 \geq \sigma_2 \geq \cdots \geq \sigma_M \geq 0$ are the singular values.

Assume further a preprocessed copy number ratio matrix $\mathbf{C} = [\mathbf{c}_1, \ldots, \mathbf{c}_M]$. Note that here we assume that the number of samples in the gene expression matrix is identical to the number of samples in the copy number ratio matrix, i.e., $M = N$. The GSVD theorem (Golub and Loan, 1996) states that for $\mathbf{E}$ and $\mathbf{C}$ there exist orthogonal matrices $\mathbf{U} \in \mathbb{R}^{m \times m}$ and $\mathbf{V} \in \mathbb{R}^{n \times n}$, and a non-singular matrix $\mathbf{X} \in \mathbb{R}^{M \times M}$ such that

$$\mathbf{U}^T \mathbf{E} \mathbf{X} = \mathrm{diag}(\alpha_1, \ldots, \alpha_M)$$

and

$$\mathbf{V}^T \mathbf{C} \mathbf{X} = \mathrm{diag}(\beta_1, \ldots, \beta_p)$$

where $p = \min(n, M)$, $\alpha_i \geq 0$ for $1 \leq i \leq M$ and $\beta_i \geq 0$ for $1 \leq i \leq p$. In practice the number of samples is much less than the number of genes on the microarray, so usually $p = M$.

In order to apply the GSVD theorem to gene expression and copy number data integration, a more general formulation of the GSVD theorem for two matrices having the same number of columns is needed. After algebraic manipulations (details are given in Berger et al., 2006) the equation for the matrix pair $\mathbf{E}$ and $\mathbf{C}$ is

$$\beta_i^2 \mathbf{E}^T \mathbf{E} \mathbf{x}_i = \alpha_i^2 \mathbf{C}^T \mathbf{C} \mathbf{x}_i,$$

where $\mathbf{x}_i$ is a generalized singular vector and represents the ith column of an invertible, but not necessarily orthogonal, matrix $\mathbf{X}$. The generalized singular values are the quotients α_i/β_i.

Let $r = \mathrm{rank}\begin{pmatrix} \mathbf{E} \\ \mathbf{C} \end{pmatrix} - \mathrm{rank}(\mathbf{C})$, $s = \mathrm{rank}(\mathbf{E}) + \mathrm{rank}(\mathbf{C}) - \mathrm{rank}\begin{pmatrix} \mathbf{E} \\ \mathbf{C} \end{pmatrix}$ and $t = \mathrm{rank}\begin{pmatrix} \mathbf{E} \\ \mathbf{C} \end{pmatrix}$. Now, from the generalized singular values, r is infinite, s is finite and non-zero, and $t - r - s$ is zero. The matrix $\mathbf{X}$ serves as a link between the input data $\mathbf{E}$ and $\mathbf{C}$. Accordingly, projecting the input data onto the columns of $\mathbf{X}$ can lead to biological interpretations based on the chosen direction of the projections of the corresponding α_i and β_i.

4.4.4.1 *'Steerable gene shaving' procedure with the GSVD* Traditionally in the SVD-based analysis, the original data are projected on a lower-dimensional subspace spanned by the eigenvectors, and clusters that are tight and separated from other clusters are identified.

In the so-called 'gene shaving' approach the genes are iteratively projected on the eigenvector that corresponds to the largest singular value and thus the highest variation in the original data. The 'gene shaving' procedure with the SVD results in a nested set of clusters based on how much the values vary in the data.

When the GSVD framework is used in the 'gene shaving' approach, the 'shaving' is done in a 'steerable' fashion based on the chosen direction of the projection.

As $\alpha_i^2 + \beta_i^2 = 1$ for $i = r+1, \ldots, r+s$, there is an angle θ_i such that $\alpha_i = \cos\theta_i$ and $\beta_i = \sin\theta_i$. Thus, we can write $\sigma_i = (1 + \tan\theta_i)/(1 - \tan\theta_i)$, and in some cases we may use the angle θ_i to represent either a generalized singular value pair or a generalized singular value (Berger et al., 2006). The angular distance between **E** and **C** is given as:

$$\theta_i = \arctan\left(\frac{\alpha_i}{\beta_i}\right) - \pi/4.$$

The angular distance indicates the relative significance of the ith gene-space projection between the data sets. An angular distance of 0 represents the case where genes are of equal significance in both data sets. An angular distance of $+\pi/4$ indicates that there is no significance in the second data set (e.g. **C**) as compared to the first (e.g. **E**), and *vice versa* for $-\pi/4$. Thus, the most interesting cases are $\theta_{\min}$, $\theta_{\max}$ and $\theta \approx 0$.

When the iterative 'steerable gene shaving' procedure is used to integrate gene expression and CGH data, the input set at each iteration is projected onto the column of **X** that corresponds to the direction of the highest variance for both inputs (determined by θ_i). In general, a fraction η (e.g. 90–95%) of the genes from **E** and **C** are retained. The iteration is repeated until the number of genes is greater than or equal to the number of samples. After iterations the 'steerable gene shaving' procedure does not result in a single gene but a fraction, such as the top 5–10% highest variant genes, for further annotation (Berger et al., 2006).

4.4.4.2 *An application of the data reduction model approach to integrate gene expression and array-CGH data* The 'steerable gene shaving' approach has been applied to the same 14 breast cancer cell lines as in Section 4.4.3.1 by Berger et al. (2006). The overlap between the genes identified with 'steerable gene shaving' and the statistical approach was 83%.

The performance for the 'steerable gene shaving' approach is strongly dependent on the quality of the data and proper preprocessing and transformations are needed prior to analysis. Thus, the GSVD is extremely sensitive to missing values. Thus, prior 'steerable gene shaving' the missing values should be either imputed or the corresponding genes discarded. A MATLAB implementation of the 'steerable gene shaving' approach is given in the supplement material for Berger et al. (2006).

4.4.5 Interpolation

If the gene expression values are obtained from different microarray formats as compared to the CGH data, the ith gene in the normalized expression data matrix **E** is not the same as the ith gene in the normalized CGH data matrix **C**. For the integrative analysis, it is important that the genes are in the same order. A solution is to interpolate either copy number or gene expression values from the data and impute these genes and values to the data matrices.

In general, interpolating copy number data points is biologically relevant, since the copy number ratio of a gene is influenced by the copy numbers of the genes located in the close vicinity. Therefore, a gene can be amplified with no biological reason due to the fact that a driver gene in the amplicon that promotes growth advantage to cancer cells is located next to this gene. Thus, for a gene having a gene expression value but not a copy number value, the interpolation could be done by giving the adjacent probes the same class label and imputing this label to the gene not having an original copy number measurement. If the adjacent probes have different labels it is challenging to estimate the label, and typically such a gene is discarded from the analysis. The same applies with the genes having copy number measurement but not gene expression value.

4.4.6 Gene annotation

Analysis for array-CGH and gene expression data typically results in a list of approximately a couple of hundred genes whose expression levels are influenced by copy number. A typical follow-up *in silico* analysis after identification of statistically significant genes with association of copy number and gene expression data is to link the resulting genes to biological processes and pathways.

Annotation methods are based on biological databases, such as Gene Ontology and pathway databases. Pathway analysis is covered in Chapters 6 and 7 in this book, and is not discussed here.

Gene Ontology (GO) is an organized framework for storing localization, interaction and functional data for genes (Ashburner *et al.*, 2000). The main objective for a GO analysis is to identify the function of a gene product. GO is a directed acyclic graph where the root node (Gene Ontology) is followed by three major categories: molecular function, biological processes, and cellular component. Each node in the GO graph can have five types of relations to its parents. The two most often used are the 'is_a' and 'part_of' relations. The 'is_a' relation means that a child node is a subclass of the parent node, whereas the 'part_of' relation means that a child node is a constituent of the parent node. For example, the GO term *chromosome* is in the part_of relation to the term *nucleus*, but *mitochondrial chromosome* is in the is_a relation to the term *chromosome*.

There exist several GO analysis methods to conduct annotation analysis, such as statistics based (Zeeberg *et al.*, 2003), combinatorial (Joslyn *et al.*, 2004) and information theoretic (Tao *et al.*, 1999). These methods can be used to identify biological processes or pathways that are enriched or repressed in the studied data set. This information can be used to prioritize genes and formulate new experiments to validate the relevance of the genes in cancers.

4.5 Conclusions

Microrrays provide high-resolution information about cancer genome and transcriptome. During the last 10 years, microarrays have been extensively applied to identify genome-wide copy number and gene expression signatures that are associated to particular pathophysiologies in cancer. Gene expression profiling has revealed novel diagnostic and prognostic subgroups and similarly, occurrence of particular genetic aberrations such as amplifications and deletions have classified tumours into specific biological or clinical subgroups. However, the influence of the somatic genetic alterations on gene expression levels have remained largely unknown until recently, when the direct integration of copy number and gene expression levels by microarrays have highlighted the impact of gene copy number alteration on gene expression. Microarrays have significantly facilitated integration of CGH and expression data by focusing on genes having altered expression due to copy number changes.

Computational methods to analyse high-throughput gene expression and copy number data are crucial in finding cancer relevant genes. The majority of the current work has been focused on developing methods that are able to identify amplified and over-expressed genes. Finding deleted and under-expressed genes is extremely important in cancer research, but currently available tools often have problems to identify such genes in a reliable manner, mainly due to the small signal-to-noise ratio. Further, several cancers have distinct characteristics, such as small copy number alterations, and to systematically detect biologically relevant regions without compromising the false positive rate is a real challenge to be addressed. Another important approach is to develop methods to further annotate the genes identified from analysis via GO or pathways so that most likely cancer-relevant genes are prioritized. Taken together, gene copy number variation causing alterations to the expression level is highly relevant in cancer genetics. Genes detected from such integrative analysis enable prioritization of the microarray data and pinpoint potential therapeutic target genes, whose role in tumorigenesis can be followed further with functional assays.

References

Altman, N.S. and Hua, J. (2006). Extending the loop design for two-channel microarray experiments. *Genetical Research*, **88**(3), 153–163.

Ashburner, M., Ball, C.A., Blake, J.A., Botstein, D., Butler, H., Cherry, J.M., Davis, A.P., Dolinski, K., Dwight, S.S., Eppig, J.T., Harris, M.A., Hill, D.P., Issel-Tarver, L., Kasarskis, A., Lewis, S., Matese, J.C., Richardson, J.E., Ringwald, M., Rubin, G.M., and Sherlock, G. (2000). Gene ontology: tool for the unification of biology. *Nature Genetics*, **25**(1), 25–29.

Autio, R., Hautaniemi, S., Kauraniemi, P., Yli-Harja, O., Astola, J., Wolf, M., and Kallioniemi, A. (2003). CGH-Plotter: MATLAB toolbox for CGH-data analysis. *Bioinformatics*, **19**(13), 1714–1715.

Berger, J.A., Hautaniemi, S., Järvinen, A.K., Edgren, H., Mitra, S.K., and Astola, J. (2004). Optimized lowess normalization parameter selection for dna microarray data. *BMC Bioinformatics*, **9**(5), 194.

Berger, J.A., Hautaniemi, S., Mitra, S.K., and Astola, J. (2006). Jointly analyzing gene expression and copy number data in breast cancer using data reduction models. *IEEE/ACM Transactions on Computational Biology and Bioinformatics*, **3**(1), 2–16.

Chen, Y., Dougherty, E., and Bittner, M. (1997). Ratio-based decisions and the quantitative analysis of cDNA microarray images. *Journal of Biomedical Optics*, **2**(4), 364–374.

References

Draghici, S. (2003). *Data Analysis for DNA Microarrays*, 2nd edn. CRC Press.

Fridlyand, J., Snijders, A.M., Pinkel, D., Albertson, D.G., and Jain, A.N. (2004). Hidden markov models approach to the analysis of array cgh data. *Journal of Multivariate Analysis*, **90**(1), 132–153.

Fridlyand, J., Snijders, A.M., Ylstra, B., Li, H., Olshen, A., Segraves, R., Dairkee, S., Tokuyasu, T., Ljung, B.M., Jain, A.N., McLennan, J., Ziegler, J., Chin, K., Devries, S., Feiler, H., Gray, J.W., Waldman, F., Pinkel, D., and Albertson, D.G. (2006). Breast tumor copy number aberration phenotypes and genomic instability. *BMC Cancer*, **6**, 96.

Golub, H.G. and Loan, C.F. Van (1996). *Matrix Computations*, 3rd edn. John Hopkins University Press.

Hautaniemi, S., Edgren, H., Vesanen, P., Wolf, M., Järvinen, A.K., Yli-Harja, O., Astola, J., Kallioniemi, O., and Monni, O. (2003). A novel strategy for microarray quality control using Bayesian networks. *Bioinformatics*, **19**(16), 2031–2038.

Hautaniemi, S., Ringnér, M., Kauraniemi, P., Autio, R., Edgren, H., Yli-Harja, O., Astola, J., Kallioniemi, A., and Kallioniemi, O.P. (2004). A strategy for identifying putative causes of gene expression variation in human cancer. *Journal of The Jefferson Institute*, **341**(1–2), 77–88.

Hyman, E., Kauraniemi, P., Hautaniemi, S., Wolf, M., Mousses, S., Rozenblum, E., Ringnér, M., Sauter, G., Monni, O., Elkahloun, A., Kallioniemi, O.P., and Kallioniemi, A. (2002). Impact of DNA amplification on gene expression patterns in breast cancer. *Cancer Research*, **62**(21), 6240–6245.

Iafrate, A.J., Feuk, L., Rivera, M.N., Listewnik, M.L., Donahoe, P.K., Qi, Y., Scherer, S.W., and Lee, C. (2004). Detection of large-scale variation in the human genome. *Nature Genetics*, **36**(9), 949–951.

Järvinen, A.K., Autio, R., Haapa-Paananen, S., Wolf, M., Saarela, M., R.G., Leivo, I., Kallioniemi, O., Mäkitie, A.A., and Monni, O. (2006). Identification of target genes in laryngeal squamous cell carcinoma by high-resolution copy number and gene expression microarray analyses. *Oncogene*, **25**, 6997–7008.

Joslyn, C.A., Mniszewski, S.M., AF, and Heaton, G. (2004). The gene ontology categorizer. *Bioinformatics*, **4**(20 Suppl 1), i169–77.

Kallioniemi, A., Kallioniemi, O.P., Sudar, D., Rutovitz, D., Gray, J.W., Waldman, F., and Pinkel, D. (1992). Comparative genomic hybridization for molecular cytogenetic analysis of solid tumors. *Science*, **258**(5083), 818–821.

Kerr, M.K. and Churchill, G.A. (2001). Experimental design for gene expression microarrays. *Biostatistics*, **2**(2), 183–201.

Knudson, A.G. (2001). Two genetic hits (more or less) to cancer. *Nature Reviews Cancer*, **1**, 157–162.

Knuutila, S., Aalto, Y., Autio, K., Bjorkqvist, A.M., El-Rifai, W., Hemmer, S., Huhta, T., Kettunen, E., Kiuru-Kuhlefelt, S., Larramendy, M.L., Lushnikova, T., Monni, O., Pere, H., Tapper, J., Tarkkanen, M., Varis, A., Wasenius, V.M., Wolf, M., and Zhu, Y. (1999). DNA copy number losses in human neoplasms. *Am. J. Pathol.*, **155**, 683–694.

Lai, W., Choudhary, V., and Park, P.J. (2008). CGHweb: a tool for comparing DNA copy number segmentations from multiple algorithms. *Bioinformatics*, **24**(7), 1014–5.

Lai, W.R., Johnson, M.D., Kucherlapati, R., and Park, P.J. (2005). Comparative analysis of algorithms for identifying amplifications and deletions in array cgh data. *Bioinformatics*, **21**(19), 3763–70.

Liang, P. and Pardee, A.B. (1992). Differential display of eukaryotic messenger RNA by means of the polymerase chain reaction. *Science*, **257**, 967–971.

Lockhart, D.J., Dong, H., Byrne, M.C., Follettie, M.T., Gallo, M.V., Chee, M.S., Mittmann, M., Wang, C., Kobayashi, M., Horton, H., and Brown, E.L. (1996). Expression monitoring by hybridization to high-density oligonucleotide arrays. *Nature Biotechnology*, **14**, 1675–1680.

Myllykangas, S., Junnila, S., Kokkola, A., Autio, R., Scheinin, I., Kiviluoto, T., Karjalainen-Lindsberg, M.L., Hollmén, J., Knuutila, S., Puolakkainen, P., and Monni, O. (2008). Integrated gene copy number and expression microarray analysis of gastric cancer highlights potential target genes. *International Journal of Cancer*, **123**(4), 817–25.

Olshen, A.B., Venkatraman, E.S., Lucito, R.L., and Wigler, M. (2004). Circular binary segmentation for the analysis of array-based DNA copy number data. *Biostatistics*, **5**(4), 557–78.

Picard, F., Robin, S., Lavielle, M., Vaisse, C., and Daudin, J.J. (2005). A statistical approach for array cgh data analysis. *BMC Bioinformatics*, **6**(6), 27.

Pinkel, D., Segraves, R., Sudar, D., Clark, S., Poole, I., Kowbel, D., Collins, C., Kuo, W.L., Chen, C., Zhai, Y., Dairkee, S.H., Ljung, B.M., Gray, J.W., and Albertson, D.G. (1998). High resolution analysis of DNA copy number variation using comparative genomic hybridization to microarrays. *Nature Genetics*, **20**, 207–211.

Pollack, J.R., Perou, C.M., Alizadeh, A.A., Eisen, M.B., Pergamenschikov, A., Williams, C.F., Jeffrey, S.S., Botstein, D., and Brown, P.O. (1999). Genome-wide analysis of DNA copy-number changes using cDNA microarrays. *Nature Genetics*, **23**(1), 41–46.

Pollack, J.R., Sorlie, T., Perou, C.M., Rees, C.A., Jeffrey, S.S., Lonning, P.E., Tibshirani, R., Botstein, D., Borresen-Dale, A.L., and Brown, P.O. (2002). Microarray analysis reveals a major direct role of DNA copy number alteration in the transcriptional program of human breast tumors. *Proceedings of the National Academy of Sciences USA*, **99**, 12963–12968.

Pollock, J.R. (2002). Gene expression profiling: methodological challenges, results, and prospects for addiction research. *Chemistry and Physics of Lipids*, **121**(1–2), 241–256.

Schena, M., Shalon, D., Davis, R.W., and Brown, P.O. (1995). Quantitative monitoring of gene expression patterns with complementary DNA microarray. *Science*, **270**(5235), 467–470.

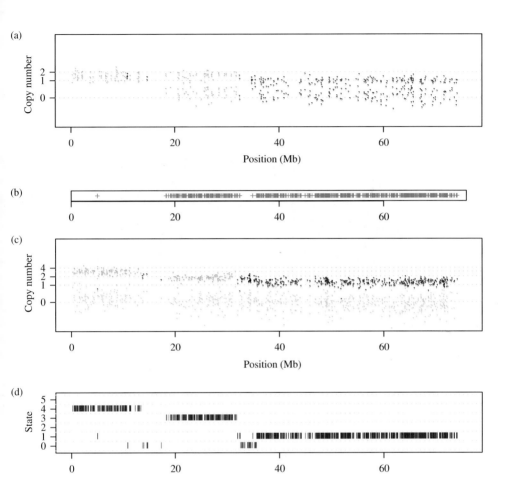

PLATE 1: An example of the HMM applied to chromosome 18 in a bladder tumour sample. In this chromosome, we can distinguish uniparental disomy coloured in purple in a region of approximatively 15 Mb and LOH in the rest of the q-arm coloured in blue. In addition, the p-arm has experienced an unbalanced amplification, coloured in orange. (a) For each SNP heterozygous in the germline DNA, the normalized intensities of each allele are plotted. The colours represent the estimated state of the SNP: black for state 0, blue for state 1, green for state 2, purple for state 3, orange for state 4 and red for state 5. (b) Shown is the region of LOH. (c) For each SNP homozygous in the germline DNA, the normalized intensities of each allele are plotted. The absent allele is coloured in grey. (d) Shown is the estimated sequence of hidden states. The colour indicates the posterior probabilities of the states: blue > 0.99, green > 0.95, orange > 0.9 and red < 0.9. See Figure 3.10 on page 73.

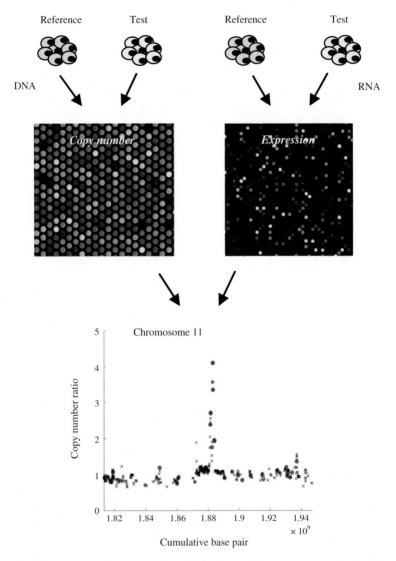

PLATE 2: To study gene expression alterations that are associated with DNA copy number alterations, DNA and RNA can be extracted from the same sample and hybridized on both the gene expression and CGH microarrays. An example of a microarray experiment, where the data has been integrated using an expression annotated copy number (ECN) tool for chromosome 11 is shown. This sample shows high-level amplication of 11q13. See Figure 4.1 on page 83.

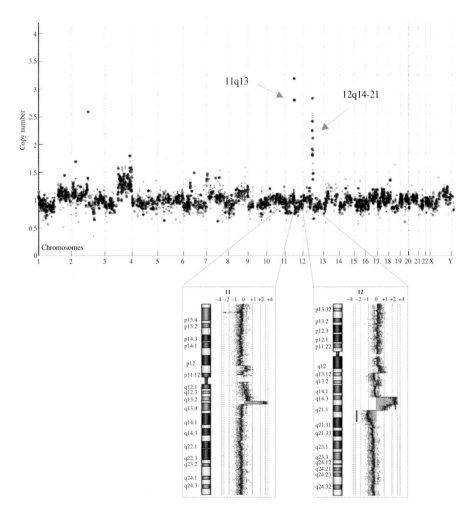

PLATE 3: Gene-expression annotated copy number plot for head and neck squamous cell carcinoma cell line. All the cDNA clones on array-CGH are arranged on the X-axis according to their base-pair position in the genome. The Y-axis shows the copy number ratio for each clone. If the ratio exceeds 1.3, the gene is regarded as amplified and if it is below 0.7, the gene is regarded as deleted. The color-coding indicates the gene expression ratio of each gene on a microarray. Red indicates over-expression, whereas green indicates under-expression. This figure illustrates that most of the genes in highly amplified regions show increased gene expression ratio. Below the expression-annotated copy number plot are shown the corresponding high-resolution copy number profiles for two highly amplified regions, 11q13 and 12q14-21, using oligonucleotide array that consists of 185,000 oligonucleotides on a single array. These views show that a number of genes are located in highly amplified regions. See Figure 4.2 on page 86.

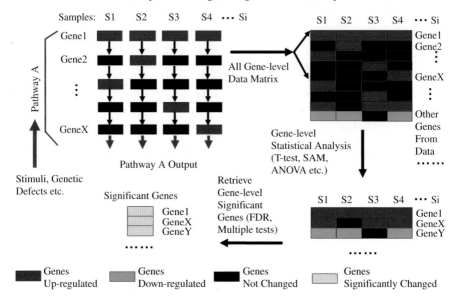
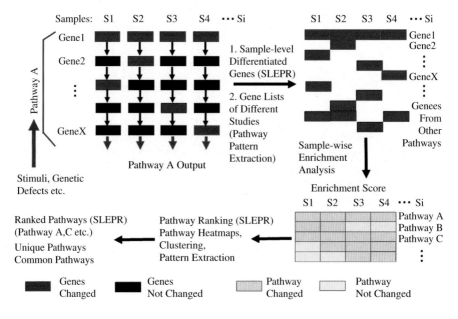

PLATE 4: Comparison of conventional gene-level methods and SLEPR or Pathway-level Pattern Extraction. Graphical display and comparison of the brief procedures for analysis using conventional gene-level methods vs. SLEPR or Pathway-level Pattern Extraction methods. Pathway A was shown as an example pathway among the whole biological system, in which many of its involved genes were changed triggered by biological stimuli, or genetic defects in disease states. The conventional gene-level methods and SLEPR or Pathway-level Pattern Extraction pipeline processed the genes from pathway A as well as other pathways in different ways even for the same biological situations under study. (a) Within a typical procedure of gene-level methods, all measured data of each sample in study are usually put together into a gene-level data matrix, and then a statistical analysis method (T-test, SAM, ANOVA, etc.) is applied to all genes of the matrix to retrieve the gene-level significant genes based on one or more statistical parameters (e.g. p-value, fold change, FDR, etc.). Significant genes usually behave with a greater gene-level consistency across samples in each population of contrasted classes. (b) For the SLEPR procedure, all measured data of each sample are used to derive the sample-level differentiated genes, which represent genes for each sample that are expressed differentiatelly compared to the rest of samples in the population (see SLEPR manuscript for details, each sample will get a corresponding list of sample-level differentiated genes). Then, sample-level differentiated genes (for SLEPR) or all gene lists of different studies (for Pathway-level Pattern Extraction pipeline) were used to perform sample-wise enrichment analysis against each of functional annotation categories (e.g. GO terms, GSEA annotation terms, or Biocarta Pathways, etc.). The derived enrichment scores (ES) of each term in the chosen functional category for each gene list were combined into an enrichment score matrix. Then pathway ranking (for SLEPR), pathway ES heatmaps, clustering, and pattern extraction (for Pathway-level Pattern Extraction) will be applied to this ES matrix to get significantly ranked pathways (SLEPR), unique pathways, common pathways (for Pathway-level Pattern Extraction), respectively. Genes that are associated with these pathways or terms can be retrieved further within the Pathway Pattern Extraction pipeline. See Figure 6.1 on page 148.

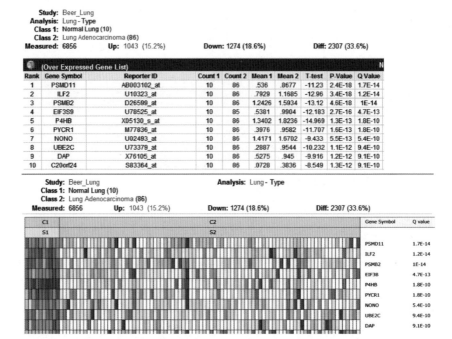

PLATE 5: Sample Differential Expression Gene List and Heat Map results from a single study (Beer_Lung) that compares gene expression in Lung Adenocarcinoma to Normal Lung in Oncomine. Genes are ranked by Q-value. See Figure 7.1 on page 162.

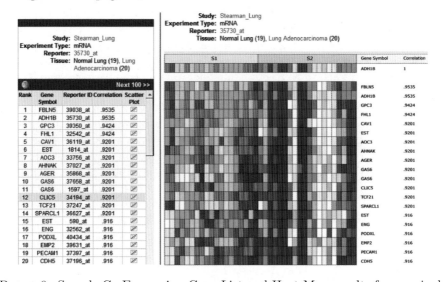

PLATE 6: Sample Co-Expression Gene List and Heat Map results from a single study (Stearman_Lung) containing Normal Lung and Lung Adenocarcinoma samples in Oncomine. The ADH1B cluster has a correlation of 0.9201 (correlation value of the 10th ranked gene) with a count size of 14 (number of genes that have a correlation of 0.9201 or better). See Figure 7.2 on page 163.

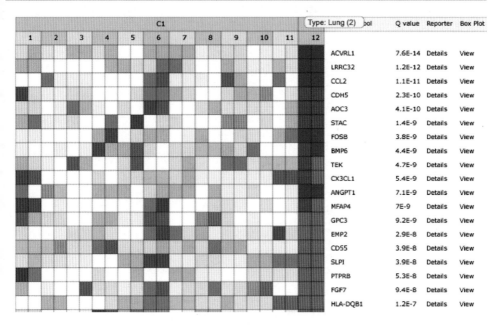

PLATE 7: Heat map of genes over-expressed in normal lung as compared to a number of other normal tissues, filtered by the set of genes identified in a meta-analysis of genes under-expressed in lung adenocarcinoma as compared to normal lung. See Figure 7.5 on page 171.

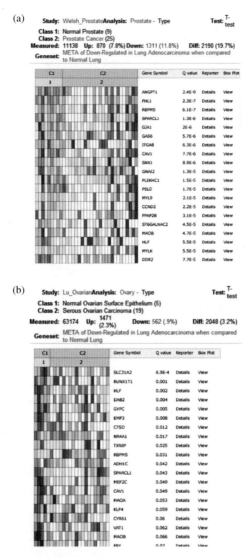

PLATE 8: Heat map of genes under-expressed in cancer as compared to normal tissues, filtered by the set of genes identified in a meta-analysis of genes under-expressed in lung adenocarcinoma as compared to normal lung. (a) Normal prostate vs. prostate cancer. (b) Normal ovary vs. ovarian carcinoma. See Figure 7.6 on page 172.

Schrock, E., du Manoir, S., Veldman, T., Schoell, B., Wienberg, J., Ferguson-Smith, M.A., Ning, Y., Ledbetter, D.H., Bar-Am, I., Soenksen, D., Garini, Y., and Ried, T. (1996). Multicolor spectral karyotyping of human chromosomes. *Science*, **273**, 494–497.

Sebat, J., Lakshmi, B., Troge, J., Alexander, J., Young, J., Lundin, P., Maner, S., Massa, H., Walker, M., Chi, M., Navin, N., Lucito, R., Healy, J., Hicks, J., Ye, K., Reiner, A., Gilliam, T.C., Trask, B., Patterson, N., Zetterberg, A., and Wigler, M. (2004). Large-scale copy number polymorphism in the human genome. *Science*, **305**(5683), 525–528.

Solinas-Toldo, S., Lampel, S., Stilgenbauer, S., Nickolenko, J., Benner, A., Dohner, H., Cremer, T., and Lichter, P. (1997). Matrix-based comparative genomic hybridization: biochips to screen for genomic imbalances. *Genes Chromosomes Cancer*, **20**, 399–407.

Tao, Y., Sam, L., Li, J., Friedman, C., and Lussier, Y.A. (1999). Information theory applied to the sparse gene ontology annotation network to predict novel gene function. *Bioinformatics*, **23**(13), i529–i538.

Velculescu, V.E., Zhang, L., Vogelstein, B., and Kinzler, K.W. (1995). Serial analysis of gene expression. *Science*, **270**, 484–487.

Wolf, M., Mousses, S., Hautaniemi, S., Karhu, R., Huusko, P., Allinen, M., Elkahloun, A., Monni, O., Chen, Y., Kallioniemi, A., and Kallioniemi, O.P. (2004). High-resolution analysis of gene copy number alterations in human prostate cancer using CGH on cDNA microarrays: impact of copy number on gene expression. *Neoplasia*, **6**(3), 240–247.

Yang, Y.H., Dudoit, S., Luu, P., and Speed, T. (2001). Normalization for cDNA microarray data. In *Microarrays: Optical Technologies and Informatics* (ed. M. Bittner, Y. Chen, A. Dorsel, and E. Dougherty), Volume 4266, pp. 141–152. SPIE.

Zeeberg, B.R., Feng, W., Wang, G., Wang, M.D., Fojo, A.T., Sunshine, M., Narasimhan, S., Kane, D.W., Reinhold, W.C., Lababidi, S., Bussey, K.J., Riss, J., Barrett, J.C., and Weinstein, J.N. (2003). Gominer: a resource for biological interpretation of genomic and proteomic data. *Genome Biology*, **4**(4), R28.

Zhang, W., Shmulevich, I., and Astola, J. (2004). *Microarray Quality Control.* Wiley-Liss.

5

ANALYSIS OF DNA METHYLATION IN CANCER

Fabian Model, Jörn Lewin, Catherine Lofton-Day and Gunter Weiss

5.1 Introduction

Sequencing genomic DNA gives the blueprint for all possible types of cells in an organism and determines the sequences that can be transcribed into mRNA and translated into proteins. RNA expression and protein analysis give a snapshot of a particular cell state at one point in time. In addition to DNA sequence information, which is constant for an individual, and the levels of generated mRNAs and proteins which vary for every cell and over time, complex organisms have another *epigenetic* layer of information.

The term *epigenetics* defines all meiotically and mitotically heritable changes in gene expression that are not coded in the DNA sequence itself. Epigenetics can, for instance, explain why the different cell types of an organism share identical DNA sequences but show broad morphological and functional diversity. Methylation of DNA is the most extensively studied of epigenetic mechanisms, and is associated with a wide range of critical biological processes. In particular it plays a fundamental role in the development of cancer.

5.1.1 DNA methylation biology

DNA methylation in vertebrates is a chemical modification of the cytosine nucleotide in which the 5-carbon position is enzymatically modified by the addition of a methyl group, such that cytosines can occur in a methylated or unmethylated state. In human DNA, methylation of cytosines occurs almost exclusively in the two-base palindromic sequence of cytosine followed by guanine, so-called *CpG*s.[1] Within a single human cell the methylation of most CpG loci can have three states: 0% homozygote unmethylated, 100% homozygote methylated or 50% heterozygote methylated.

The CpG dinucleotide is underrepresented in the human genome, likely because methylated cytosines are prone to deamination producing thymine, resulting in a G/T mismatch. This mutagenic property is postulated to have driven CpG depletion during evolution. Most of the CpG dinucleotides in the human genome are methylated (between 60 and 70%). However, CpG rich clusters of between three hundred and several thousand base pairs, so-called CpG islands, are found close to the 5′ regulatory regions of many genes and are generally not methylated. CpG islands that have a majority of their CpG dinucleotides

---

[1]*CpG* means *C*ytosine, *p*hosphate bound, *G*uanine. The sequence is palindromic: it is identical to its reverse complement.

unmethylated are referred to as *hypomethylated* whereas islands with a majority of methylated CpGs are called *hypermethylated*.

Hypermethylation of a CpG island is usually associated with transcriptional silencing of the neighbouring gene. The symmetrical addition of the methyl group changes the appearance of the major groove of the double helix and directly influences transcription by altering the binding of sequence specific transcription factors, repressors, and insulators (Ehrlich, 2003). An indirect reinforcement of the transcriptionally silent state is mediated by proteins that can bind to methylated CpGs. These proteins, which are called methyl-CpG binding proteins, recruit histone deacetylases and other chromatin remodelling proteins that can modify histones, thereby forming compact, inactive chromatin termed heterochromatin (Hendrich and Tweedie, 2003). However, methylation does not cause transcriptional silencing in every case. When a negative regulatory element such as a silencer is hypermethylated expression of the associated gene can actually increase.

DNA methylation has been shown to play a key role in the following genetic mechanisms: tissue differentiation, silencing of repetitive elements and endogenous transposons, X chromosome inactivation in females, inactivation of one allele in parent-of-origin specific manner (imprinting), and interaction between gene activation and environment.

DNA methylation is maintained and propagated to new cell generations by DNA methyl transferases (DNMT). The exact mechanism of how methylation patterns are initially established during implantation of the zygote and later regulated is still unknown. However, one can observe that methylation states of adjacent CpG dinucleotides are highly correlated and that methylation signatures of different cell types vary in *co-methylated* blocks of a few hundred base pairs (Eckhardt et al., 2006). This observation implies that mechanisms for methylation and de-methylation address whole blocks of co-methylated CpG dinucleotides which are likely associated with one biological function.

5.1.2 DNA methylation in cancer

DNA methylation plays an important role in several human diseases but is probably most extensively studied in cancer. In virtually all types of human carcinoma dramatic changes of DNA methylation patterns have been reported for tumours compared to normal tissues. The most common alterations are a genome wide hypomethylation and gene specific hypermethylation. Genome wide hypomethylation mainly affects repetitive sequences in satellite DNA and centromeres causing a general loss of genome stability.

Silencing of tumour suppressor genes by promoter hypermethylation usually affects genes involved in DNA repair, detoxification, cell cycle regulation, or apoptosis (Jones and Baylin, 2002). Knudson's two hit hypothesis postulates that for the development of a malignant cell both alleles of a tumour suppressor gene have to be inactivated. Promoter hypermethylation leading to gene silencing can be one of those hits. Together with other events like mutation or loss of heterozygosity (LOH) promoter hypermethylation can completely deactivate a tumour suppressor gene and cause malignancy of a cell (Grady et al., 2000).

Since in contrast to genetic mutations, epigenetic alterations of tumour DNA are potentially reversible they could be interesting targets for future therapeutics (Egger et al., 2004). An application of DNA methylation that is realizable in the near future is the development of biomarkers for diagnosis of cancer. In particular the hypermethylation of specific tumour suppressor genes has considerable advantages compared to tumour markers based on analysis of somatic mutations, mRNA expression or proteins: (1) Promoter hypermethylation occurs early in tumorigenesis and can be specific for certain tumour types. (2) Hypermethylation of certain genes does not exist in normal cells. For these markers hypermethylation is a distinct qualitative and specific sign of malignancy and can be detected in a background of normal cells with high sensitivity. (3) Compared to mRNA and protein measurements methylation patterns are very stable over time. (4) Methylation can be quantified in relation to the total amount of DNA. This enables easy comparison between different measurements. (5) In contrast to somatic mutations (such as single nucleotide polymorphisms (SNPs)) DNA methylation signals occur at distinct and well defined genomic locations.

Therefore DNA methylation analysis can be used for a variety of applications in cancer diagnosis. One is the classification of tissue samples taken either from a biopsy of a suspicious lesion or from a surgically removed tumour (Adorjan et al., 2002). Typical diagnostic questions that have to be answered based on these tissue samples are: (1) Malignancy – Is the tumour benign or malignant? (2) Prognosis – How aggressive is the tumour? Will the patient have a relapse after surgery? (3) Prediction of therapy response – How will the tumour respond to a certain treatment? Is a particular chemotherapy necessary?

Technically, fresh frozen or paraffin embedded tissue samples are the optimal source material for methylation analysis since they provide sufficient amounts of DNA that comes almost completely from the tumour tissue of interest. The disadvantage is that these samples usually require an invasive procedure that carries a certain risk, is unpleasant for the patient and of course that the tumour has to be actually diagnosed and located.

Another application of DNA methylation analysis is the detection of cancer in remote samples. Due to their uncontrolled growth and high rate of cell necrosis tumours can shed relatively high amounts of their DNA into body fluids such as blood or urine. By using sensitive detection methods that can identify methylated tumour DNA biomarkers in an excess of normal DNA, it is possible to diagnose cancer based on a simple blood or urine test (Lofton-Day et al., 2008). This kind of analysis does not require an invasive procedure, is very convenient for the patient, and therefore promises a high compliance in screening programs aimed at asymptomatic populations.[2]

---

[2] A disease is asymptomatic when the patient does not experience any noticeable symptoms. This is typical for early stage cancers. They can only be diagnosed by systematically screening an entire population, including a vast majority of healthy individuals.

A third application of DNA methylation in cancer diagnostics is the identification of patients that are at risk of developing a cancer over the course of their lives. This kind of predisposition can be caused by a loss of imprinting (LOI). An example is the gene *Insulin Growth Factor II* (IGF2) that is usually methylated on the maternal allele, resulting in expression of only the paternal allele. The loss of maternal imprinting is found in children with Wilm's tumours and it has been shown that loss of IGF2 imprinting increases the risk of developing colorectal cancer. Since LOI is a defect that arises during germline development, it is present in all patient cells and can be conveniently detected in blood (Cui et al., 2003).

5.1.3 Overview

In the following sections we will give a short overview of technologies used for measuring DNA methylation and discuss how it can be quantified. We will take a more detailed look at data pre-processing algorithms for two of the most commonly used high-throughput measurement technologies: direct bisulphite DNA sequencing and DNA methylation microarrays. Then we will show some typical examples for DNA methylation data analysis in cancer research: the classification of tissue samples, the detection of cancer in plasma samples, and the prediction of tumour recurrence. Finally we will give a short summary and conclusions.

5.2 Measuring DNA methylation

All of the technologies used for measuring DNA methylation originate either from DNA sequence or mRNA expression analysis. However, the technology transfer is not trivial. In contrast to the basic sequence of the DNA, its methylation patterns vary from cell to cell. This makes methylation analysis of tissue or body fluid samples inherently quantitative. On the other hand DNA methylation patterns are limited to a finite number of CpG methylation state permutations within the given set of cells. In contrast to expression analysis the concentrations of these sequence variants are very much constrained since they are merely proportions of the total DNA in the sample. Due to these fundamental differences the respective technologies and the interpretation of the raw measurement values have to be substantially modified.

5.2.1 Measurement technologies

For the analysis of DNA methylation, sensitive and quantitative methods are needed to detect even subtle changes in the degree of methylation, as biological samples often represent a heterogeneous mixture of different cells, e.g. tumour and non-tumour cells. A variety of techniques for the study of DNA methylation have been developed over the last few years (Fraga and Esteller, 2002; Laird, 2003). All methods have different advantages and disadvantages with regard to quantitative accuracy, sensitivity, genome coverage and precise investigations of individual CpG positions (see Fig. 5.1). Therefore the choice of method mainly depends on the desired application. DNA methylation measurement techniques can be roughly classified into methods analysing the total amount of

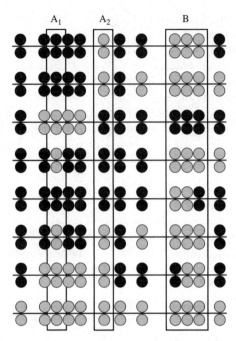

FIG. 5.1: Principles of DNA methylation analysis. A genomic DNA sample usually consists of a heterogeneous mix of DNA molecules derived from many different cells. In this figure, each horizontal bar represents an entire double stranded haploid genome. Eight such haploid genomes are aligned above each other. Circles represent cytosine residues in the context of CpG dinucleotides on the top or bottom strand of the DNA double helix. Methylated cytosines are represented by black circles, unmethylated cytosines by grey circles. DNA methylation analysis methods measure either each individual CpG methylation status (cloned bisulphite sequencing), the proportion of methylated cytosines at one CpG position, e.g. the relative number of black dots in columns A_1 and A_2 (methylation sensitive restriction methods, direct bisulphite sequencing, MeDIP), the proportion of specific cytosine methylation patterns at one set of CpG positions, e.g. the relative number of completely methylated black blocks in columns B (MSP, bisulphite microarrays), or the overall amount of cytosine methylation, i.e. the total number of black dots (global methylation analysis). Note that the methylation proportion estimates for columns A_1 and A_2 are identical even though the respective methylation events occur in different cells.

methylcytosine in a sample, methods based on enrichment of methylated DNA by immunoprecipitation, methods based on methylation sensitive enzymatic digestion of genomic DNA, and methods relying on bisulphite conversion.

One of the most widely used techniques for the monitoring of global changes in methylation levels is HPLC following a quantitative hydrolysis of the DNA sample to single nucleotides. Increased sensitivity with smaller amounts of DNA can be achieved by capillary electrophoresis or mass spectrometry. *In situ* hybridization methods with methylcytosine specific antibodies can be used to specifically target methylated sequences allowing detection of methylation on a cell to cell basis. However, since global methylation analysis is per definition completely unspecific with regard to genomic location it is not usable for most diagnostic purposes.

Methylcytosine specific antibodies can also be used in combination with an immunocapturing approach to measure methylation at specific CpG positions within the genome. When the genomic DNA is randomly sheared and immunoprecipitated to enrich for methylated DNA fragments (methylated DNA immunoprecipitation, or MeDIP), the methylation rate at a specific CpG position can be determined, e.g. by hybridization of the enriched DNA to a DNA tiling microarray (Weber et al., 2005).

Traditionally methylation patterns have been analysed by digestion of genomic DNA with methylation sensitive restriction endonucleases and subsequent detection by Southern blotting or PCR amplification. A variety of methods have been developed that use the restriction digest of DNA with methylation sensitive enzymes to compare genome wide methylation patterns between two samples or two pools of samples. Prominent examples are restriction landmark genomic scanning, CpG island amplification, methylation sensitive arbitrarily primed PCR and differential methylation hybridization (DMH) (Yan et al., 2000). The DMH methodology in combination with high-density single colour DNA microarrays can also be used for an absolute quantification of methylation rates on a genome wide scale (Lewin et al., 2007). The fundamental limitation of all these methylation sensitive restriction enzyme based technologies is their dependence on the presence of restriction sites in the sequence containing the CpG sites of interest.

The introduction of sodium bisulphite conversion of genomic DNA has revolutionized the field of DNA methylation analysis. Bisulphite treatment of genomic DNA samples results in the hydrolytic deamination of non-methylated cytosines to uracils, while methylated cytosines are resistant to conversion. After PCR amplification the methylation status at a given position is manifested in the ratio C (former methylated cytosine) to T (former non-methylated cytosine) and can be analysed as a virtual C/T polymorphism in the bisulphite treated DNA.

A commonly applied method for the assessment of the methylation status is either direct sequencing or sequencing of subclones of bisulphite treated DNA (Frommer et al., 1992). It is so far the only method that allows a thorough analysis of multiple, closely neighbouring CpG positions. Cloned bisulphite sequencing can be regarded as the gold standard of methylation analysis since it enables the measurement of the methylation status of every individual CpG dinucleotide in a sample (see Fig. 5.1). However, cloning is extremely labour intensive and costly and thus not suitable for large numbers of samples or genomic locations. Direct bisulphite sequencing can be used to measure the proportions of methylated CpG dinucleotides at a specific location and is an efficient alternative.

A high throughput method for bisulphite based methylation measurement is hybridization of bisulphite converted DNA onto microarrays (Adorjan et al., 2002; Bibikova et al., 2006). In this technology selected genes are amplified by multiplex or universally primed PCR from bisulphite treated DNA, fluorescently labelled and hybridized onto a microarray with specific oligonucleotides. Each of these detection oligonucleotides is designed to hybridize to the bisulphite converted sequence around a specific CpG site which was originally either unmethylated or methylated. Oligonucleotide hybridization intensities can then be used to derive the proportion of methylated CpG dinucleotides at the respective genomic locations.

Another popular method for the analysis of bisulphite converted DNA is methylation-specific PCR (MSP). It permits the amplification of small blocks of CpG sites with primers complementary to the methylation pattern of interest. The main advantage of MSP is the high sensitivity that enables the detection of the target allele in the presence of a huge excess of other alleles and the detection of differentially methylated positions in body fluids. Quantitation in a variable background is difficult due to the biased amplification and can be improved by fluorescence based real-time PCR assays such as MethyLight (Eads et al., 2000) or HeavyMethyl (Cottrell et al., 2004).

5.2.2 Quantification of DNA methylation

As shown in Fig. 5.1 DNA methylation signatures can be different for each individual cell. However, when we study tissue samples we are interested in methylation patterns that are characteristic for a certain tissue, e.g. a block of CpG positions that becomes hypermethylated in the majority of cancer cells but is hypomethylated in normal cells. Therefore for the study of tissue samples an analysis of the proportion of methylated CpG dinucleotides at a certain position is usually sufficient.

We define the amount of extracted DNA, N^{DNA}, as the number of DNA strands available for analysis. For a given CpG position p a certain number $N_p^{\mathrm{DNA}+}$ of strands will be methylated and a certain number $N_p^{\mathrm{DNA}-}$ will be unmethylated. Independent of the CpG position p their sum is always the total amount of DNA, $N^{\mathrm{DNA}} = N_p^{\mathrm{DNA}+} + N_p^{\mathrm{DNA}-}$. Note that the two complementary DNA strands from the same allele have identical methylation. Depending on which DNA strand the applied detection technology measures we count only 3' or 5' strands, or both.

What we want to estimate from our DNA sample is the methylation rate M_p, the proportion of methylated DNA at CpG position p. Given our DNA sample the obvious way to estimate M_p is to simply compute the proportion of methylated DNA

$$M_p = \frac{N_p^{\mathrm{DNA}+}}{N^{\mathrm{DNA}}} = 1 - \frac{N_p^{\mathrm{DNA}-}}{N^{\mathrm{DNA}}} = \frac{N_p^{\mathrm{DNA}+}}{N_p^{\mathrm{DNA}+} + N_p^{\mathrm{DNA}-}}. \tag{5.1}$$

Note that for M values to be representative for a certain tissue the DNA has to be extracted from tissue samples of high purity.

Because M is a proportion its values are restricted to a $[0\%, 100\%]$ interval. Measurement distributions on this scale are often highly skewed since the biological relevance of differences is not constant. For example a difference between $M_A = 0.1\%$ and $M_B = 10\%$ means there are a hundred times more cells that show a methylation phenotype in sample B as compared to sample A. On the other hand the same 10% difference between $M_A = 40\%$ and $M_B = 50\%$ can be easily explained by a slight difference in tissue composition. In general the closer a differential methylation rate is to the extremes of 0% or 100% the more biological relevance it has. For analysis it is often more convenient to use a scale where differences have constant relevance. This can be achieved by using the log methylation odds defined as

$$\log O_p = \log \frac{M_p}{1 - M_p} = \log \frac{N_p^{\text{DNA}+}}{N_p^{\text{DNA}-}}. \quad (5.2)$$

A difference between two log methylation odds corresponds to the log odds ratio of the two methylation rates. As a measure of methylation distance it is often more meaningful than a difference of methylation proportions.

When we measure DNA methylation in remote samples (i.e. we want to detect the presence of cancer DNA shed by a solid tumour in a body fluid like blood or urine), we require the target analyte to be completely unmethylated at the analyzed CpG positions. What we are interested in is the presence and concentration of methylated DNA from a primary tumour. Sources of methylated and unmethylated DNA are completely independent, therefore computation of a methylation rate is meaningless. The measurement value used for analysis is simply the concentration of methylated DNA. Using the logarithm of concentration measurements helps to get distances with constant relevance and symmetrical distributions.

5.3 Data preprocessing

The goal of preprocessing is to estimate DNA methylation rates from observed raw measurement values. Even though the detection technologies used to measure DNA methylation are very similar to methodologies used in DNA sequencing or expression analysis the interpretation of the raw data is completely different. Compared to classical DNA sequencing electropherogram data has to be interpreted in a quantitative way and not only qualitatively. In contrast to expression analysis, the well-defined extreme target concentrations with all or none of the CpG positions being methylated span a natural scale for quantification and enable straightforward normalization. The following sections give a short description of preprocessing algorithms for two of the most commonly used high throughput measurement technologies: direct bisulphite DNA sequencing and DNA methylation microarrays.

5.3.1 Direct bisulphite sequencing

Sequencing large numbers of subclones from a bisulphite converted DNA sample results in accurate and complete determination of methylation status on a single DNA strand level. However, this approach is labour intensive and in most cases a determination of the methylation rate at a specific CpG position is entirely sufficient. The direct sequencing of bisulphite DNA samples and the quantitative interpretation of sequencing signal intensities is a more efficient alternative that still provides quantitative methylation measurements in single CpG resolution (Lewin et al., 2004).

Quantitative methylation analysis by direct sequencing of PCR products from bisulphite treated DNA poses several challenges: poor signal quality compared to genomic sequencing, overscaled cytosine signals and basecaller artefacts. In combination with the overscaled signals incomplete bisulphite conversion might influence signal proportions in the trace.

Electropherogram data is stored in trace files and in general represented as time series of signals from the four bases A, C, G and T. The data include annotations interpreted by basecaller software: maxima of signals and the resulting DNA sequence of the sequencing experiment. One established format for trace data is the scf file format (Dear and Staden, 1992). The following algorithm is optimized for four dye electropherogram trace file data pre-processed by standard basecaller software (e.g. from Applied Biosystems).

The data processing includes the following steps: (1) entropy based clipping, (2) signal detection, (3) alignment, (4) trace correction, (5) alignment based clipping, (6) equalization of signal intensities, (7) signal normalization, and (8) compensation of incomplete conversion and methylation estimation. The algorithm assumes forward sequencing and aims at estimating the proportion of cytosine to thymine at the positions of interest. Traces that originate from reverse sequencing and show guanine and adenine signals can be analysed in the same way by building the reverse complement of the trace files.

5.3.1.1 Entropy based clipping

We observed that basecallers often generate reads that contain long stretches of called bases with up-scaled background signals after the end of an amplificate. These artefacts are detected by using the Shannon entropy

$$H = -\sum_{b \in B} \frac{S_b}{\sum_{b' \in B} S_{b'}} \log_4 \frac{S_b}{\sum_{b' \in B} S_{b'}} \qquad (5.3)$$

of the four trace curves S_b, where b and b' stand for one of the four bases $B = \{A, C, G, T\}$. The entropy is calculated in a sliding window of 200 data points in the time series space of the trace signal data. Flanking sequence stretches with an entropy larger than 0.8 are removed.

5.3.1.2 Signal detection

For each base position in the trace file we compute the corresponding intensities $A^{\text{int}}, C^{\text{int}}, G^{\text{int}}, T^{\text{int}}$ that estimate the base proportions

Data preprocessing

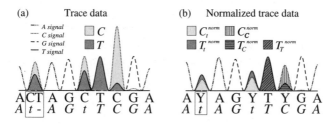

FIG. 5.2: Schematic representation of a trace file electropherogram obtained by bisulphite PCR sequencing (a) before and (b) after signal normalization. The upper sequences below the trace curves in (a) represent the sequence called by the standard basecaller and in (b) the peak mixture represented using IUPAC code. The sequences at the bottom show the aligned reference sequence. The lower case t stands for genomic cytosine positions that are not in CpG context. Since they are unmethylated they should be converted to thymine after bisulphite treatment and PCR amplification. Trace curves are shown for all four bases. For every base position in the reference sequence four base intensities $A^{\text{int}}, C^{\text{int}}, G^{\text{int}}, T^{\text{int}}$ are calculated as the area under the trace curve segment that belongs to the base position (only C and T shown in (a)). Normalized base intensities for cytosine ($C_b^{\text{norm}}; b \in \{t, C\}$) and thymine ($T_b^{\text{norm}}; b \in \{t, T, C\}$) seen in (b) are used to estimate the bisulphite conversion rate (base intensities at t positions) and the methylation level at each CpG (base intensities at C positions).

in the molecular mixture (see Fig. 5.2a). As an appropriate measure we have chosen the areas under the trace (S_b) corresponding to the respective base for each position in the sequence. By default, the trace segment between neighbouring local minima is used for the signal area estimation. If no local minima are present, then the boundaries of the trace segment are estimated as the midpoint between two neighbouring inflection points.

5.3.1.3 *Alignment* The base intensities estimated in the previous step are mapped to an underlying genomic reference sequence. The *a priori* availability of the genomic sequence is a prerequisite for our application. To describe the bisulphite converted DNA, the commonly used genomic alphabet (A,C,G,T) is extended by one letter, the lower case t, to distinguish a thymine derived from cytosine by bisulphite conversion and PCR from a thymine that was present already in the genomic sequence. As an exception, cytosines in a CpG context in the reference sequence are denoted by C because their methylation status and therefore their conversion status is unknown. We use the Smith–Waterman algorithm (Barton, 1993) for optimal local alignments allowing for gaps to align the called sequence of the trace file with the *a priori* known reference sequence.

Bisulphite treated DNA contains long stretches of T signal. In some cases this is misinterpreted by basecallers by inserting too many Ts into the called sequence.

Accounting for this special situation, we have introduced a content dependent gap cost between C and G in the reference sequence that forces the alignment of CpGs as one functional block to avoid their mismapping. An example of this is given below. Costs for regular gaps are -19 and costs for gaps between C and G in the reference sequence are -39.

```
trace       ATTTTTTTGA           ATTTTTTTGA
reference   ATTTTTC-GA           ATTTTT-CGA
            cost = -39           cost = -19
```

5.3.1.4 Trace correction Standard basecallers expect one homogeneous DNA population to be sequenced, therefore they often interpret mixed C and T base intensities at a single position of the reference sequence as two adjacent bases. In contrast to standard sequencing, in our experiments we expect signal mixtures from different DNA populations. It follows that the separation of overlaying intensities belonging to one position into two bases by the basecaller has to be corrected. We identify the separated base intensities by searching adjacent T and C positions in the called sequence from which one is aligned with t or C and the other is introducing a gap into the reference sequence. These base pairs in the called sequence are then fused into a single base.

5.3.1.5 Alignment based clipping The quality of trace files from PCR product sequencing, especially of amplificates from bisulphite treated template containing different molecule populations, is lower than sequences from a homogeneous clone template. Alignment quality as a natural measure to assess sequencing quality is used to identify areas of poor quality. Flanking regions of the sequence are clipped such that the remaining inner part has less than 10% alignment error to the reference sequence.

5.3.1.6 Equalization of signal intensities Signal intensities in trace data decrease with progression of sampling time. If signals from cytosine in and out of CpG context and thymidine signals are not randomly distributed within an examined region, the proportions of those signals can be over- or under-interpreted in normalization based on accumulation at locations with extreme signal intensity. We therefore equalize all signal intensities prior to normalization by dividing all four time series of base signals $S_b(t); b \in \{A, C, G, T\}$ at each data point by the average signal intensity within a window of n data points and multiplying by 10,000:

$$S'_b(t) = S_b(t) \frac{10{,}000 n}{\sum_{b \in \{A,C,G,T\}} \sum_{i=t-n/2}^{t+n/2} S_b(i)}. \tag{5.4}$$

5.3.1.7 Signal normalization We found that cytosine trace curves are often overscaled in direct bisulphite sequencing traces. Base proportion calculation based on trace curves with different baseline intensities would give misleading results. Therefore we normalize the trace curves prior to calculating the proportions of base intensities to determine bisulphite conversion and methylation rate (Fig. 5.2b). The normalized base intensities are denoted by $A_b^{\text{norm}}, C_b^{\text{norm}}, G_b^{\text{norm}}, T_b^{\text{norm}}$; $b \in \{C, t, T\}$ and fulfil the following constraints based on average base intensities:

$$\overline{T_T^{\text{norm}}} \equiv \overline{T_C^{\text{norm}} + C_C^{\text{norm}}} \tag{5.5}$$

$$\overline{T_T^{\text{norm}}} \equiv \overline{T_t^{\text{norm}} + C_t^{\text{norm}}}. \tag{5.6}$$

The constraints simply require that after normalization thymine signals at genomic T positions should have the same average intensity as the sum of thymine and cytosine signals at genomic C positions. The first constraint states this for C positions in CpG context, the second constraint for other C positions.

Normalization of C^{int} is performed by multiplication of a global factor F_C:

$$C_b^{\text{norm}} = F_C C_b^{\text{int}}; b \in \{C, t, A, G, T\}. \tag{5.7}$$

Based on the data we use different strategies for normalization. If there are at least three C positions with $C_C^{\text{int}} > T_C^{\text{int}}$ normalization is based on eqn (5.5) with data from these positions:

$$F_C = \frac{\overline{T_T^{\text{int}} - T_C^{\text{int}}}}{\overline{C_C^{\text{int}}}}. \tag{5.8}$$

Otherwise normalization is based on eqn (5.6) with data from all t positions:

$$F_C = \frac{\overline{T_T^{\text{int}} - T_t^{\text{int}}}}{\overline{C_t^{\text{int}}}}. \tag{5.9}$$

In rare cases when all cytosines were unmethylated and converted completely ($C_C^{\text{int}} = 0$) normalization of the cytosine trace curve is impossible and unnecessary.

5.3.1.8 Compensation of incomplete conversion and methylation estimation

Cytosine base intensity at CpG positions can arise from two sources: from a population of methylated cytosines in the sample DNA and from an incomplete conversion reaction. It follows that the bisulphite conversion rate has to be first estimated to obtain a correct estimation of the methylation rate in the sample DNA. For an individual t the conversion rate R is estimated by

$$R = \frac{T_t^{\text{norm}}}{T_t^{\text{norm}} + C_t^{\text{norm}}}. \tag{5.10}$$

Local R_{loc} and global conversion rates R_{glob} can be determined by averaging over R of individual bases within defined ranges. Then the methylation rate

$M, 0 \leq M \leq 1$, at a certain CpG can be estimated by using the following simple linear relationship

$$T_C^{\text{norm}} = R_{\text{glob}}(1 - M)(T_C^{\text{norm}} + C_C^{\text{norm}}). \tag{5.11}$$

The equation describes the fact that the T base intensity at a C position T_C^{norm} is expected to arise from the unmethylated portion of the sample DNA that is bisulphite converted by rate R. Furthermore the sum of the base intensities $T_C^{\text{norm}} + C_C^{\text{norm}}$ is assumed to be proportional to the total of cytosines in the sample DNA. It follows that the methylation rate can be estimated by incorporating a correction for the incomplete bisulphite conversion as

$$M = 1 - \frac{T_C^{\text{norm}}}{(C_C^{\text{norm}} + T_C^{\text{norm}})R_{\text{glob}}}. \tag{5.12}$$

Signal variance, artefacts, or errors in the normalization might lead to negative methylation estimation which is set to 0.

5.3.2 DNA microarrays

DNA microarrays allow the concentration measurement of thousands of target sequences in parallel. Their raw measurement values are signal intensities of individual oligomer probe spots that match a specific sequence in the target DNA. Higher target sequence concentrations result in higher signal intensities. Two popular methodologies for measuring DNA methylation with microarrays are the restriction enzyme based DMH approach (Lewin et al., 2007) and bisulphite based microarray workflows (Adorjan et al., 2002; Bibikova et al., 2006).

The DMH technology works as follows. First sample DNA is cut by methylation unspecific restriction enzymes into well-defined DNA fragments and PCR priming sites are ligated. Then unmethylated fragments are cut by restriction enzymes specific for unmethylated CpG sites. Only the uncut completely methylated fragments are then amplified by PCR and fluorescently labelled. The resulting PCR product is hybridized onto a microarray with detection probes that match the fragments expected from the first methylation unspecific restriction step. Measurement probes are designed for fragments that contain methylation specific restriction sites. These measurement probes will show low signals if their matching fragment was unmethylated and high signals if their matching fragment was completely methylated. A smaller number of control probes is designed for fragments without methylation specific restriction sites. These probes will always show maximum signal intensities and can be used for normalization.

Bisulphite microarrays work as follows. First sample DNA is bisulphite converted and a selected set of DNA fragments is amplified by PCR and fluorescently labelled. The resulting PCR product is hybridized onto a microarray with detection probes that match fragment locations containing at least one CpG dinucleotide. Usually there are always two variants of each probe. The methylation detection probe matches the bisulphite sequence of a completely methylated fragment (cytosines are not converted) and the non-methylation detection probe matches the bisulphite sequence of a completely unmethylated fragment (cytosines are all converted to thymidine). Depending on the methylation status of the respective fragment the methylation or the non-methylation probe will show higher signal intensities.

The basic preprocessing steps of methylation microarray analysis are identical to classical expression microarray analysis. Algorithms for image processing, background correction, and within-array normalization are well established (Stekel, 2003) and will not be further discussed here. However, the last two preprocessing stages of between-array normalization and measurement value estimation can be performed more efficiently than in expression analysis by using specific properties of DNA methylation.

5.3.2.1 *Between-array normalization* In order to analyse expression or methylation microarray data one has to compare hybridization intensities between different arrays. Typically experimental conditions between hybridization reactions vary slightly and cause differences in the overall signal intensity of different arrays. The simplest method to correct for these differences is to scale the signal intensities of each array a by a constant factor f_a. Normalized intensities are then computed as $I_{p,a}^n = (1/f_a)I_{p,a}^r$, where p is a probe index and I^r is the original raw intensity.[3]

For expression microarrays the scaling factor f_a is classically calculated as the mean or median intensity over all probes for each individual array. This approach makes the central assumption that the variations in the signal intensity distributions between arrays are a result of experimental conditions and not biological variability. Especially when comparing drastically different cell types such as normal and cancerous tissue this assumption is obviously violated and poses a fundamental problem for expression microarray analysis. Fortunately for methylation microarrays we can use the fact that we only want to measure the proportion of methylated DNA and not its absolute concentration. This enables us to normalize each array by some measure of total DNA while retaining the relevant information for calculating the methylation rate.

In the case of the restriction enzyme based DMH microarrays we can use the signal intensities of the control probes for normalization. Since these probes are designed for fragments without methylation specific restriction sites they measure the DNA concentration in the sample independent of methylation at different genetic loci. The array normalization factor can be simply computed as the median control probe intensity:

$$f_a = \text{median}_{p \in \mathcal{C}}(I_{p,a}^r), \tag{5.13}$$

---

[3]Note that we use the same symbol p for CpG positions and probes since there is usually a one-to-one relationship between the two.

where $\mathcal{C}$ is the set of control probe indices on the used microarray layout. After normalization the control probe intensities on all arrays will be approximately identical and measurement probe intensities represent the concentrations of methylated DNA relative to total DNA.

In the case of bisulphite microarrays we can use the property that all measured CpG positions are queried by a methylation and a non-methylation detection probe. These probes show an inverse hybridization behaviour for different amounts of methylated DNA in the target sample. The methylation probe intensity increases with higher degrees of methylation; the non-methylation probe intensity decreases. As a result the sum of methylation and non-methylation probe intensity is approximately constant and independent of the degree of methylation at the respective CpG position. Therefore the array normalization factor can be computed as the median of the pairwise sum of all detection probe pairs:

$$f_a = \text{median}_p(I_{p,a}^{r+} + I_{p,a}^{r-}), \tag{5.14}$$

where I^{r+} is the raw signal intensity of the methylation detection probes, I^{r-} is the raw signal intensity of the non-methylation detection probes, and p is a probe pair index. After normalization the pairwise sum of methylation and non-methylation detection probe intensities on all arrays will be approximately identical and individual probe intensities represent the concentrations of methylated and unmethylated DNA relative to total DNA.

5.3.2.2 *Methylation rate estimation* We assume the following simple linear model to explain the observed detection probe hybridization intensities on a microarray:

$$I_p = k_p M_p + I_p^0, \tag{5.15}$$

where I_p is the expected hybridization intensity, k_p is the dynamic range of probe p (the change in hybridization intensity for a methylation change of 100%), M_p is the methylation rate at CpG position p and I_p^0 is the unmethylated background intensity of probe p. We chose here a simplified annotation that uses the same index p for CpG positions and probes assuming a one to one relation. For DMH microarrays CpG position p actually describes a particular fragment containing one or more individual CpG dinucleotides. The methylation rate M_p is in this case the proportion of completely methylated copies of fragment p. For bisulphite microarrays CpG position p refers to a set of one or more CpG dinucleotides covered by a methylation and a non-methylation detection probe. In this case eqn (5.15) actually splits into a model for the methylation detection probe $I_p^+ = k_p^+ M_p + I_p^{0+}$ and a model for the non-methylation detection probe $I_p^- = k_p^- M_p + I_p^{0-}$, each with their own parameters for dynamic range and unmethylated background intensity. Note that the slope of the linear model k_p will be positive for methylation detection and negative for non-methylation detection probes. Figure 5.3 gives a visualization of the hybridization model.

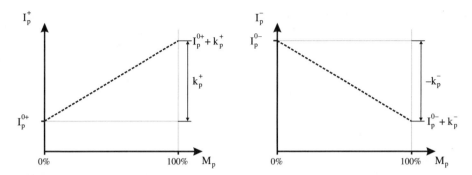

FIG. 5.3: Simple hybridization intensity model. The plots show the linear dependence between hybridization intensities and DNA methylation rate for methylation detection (left) and non-methylation detection (right) probes on a bisulphite microarray. The hybridization model for DMH microarrays is identical to the methylation detection probe model (left).

In order to estimate methylation rates from observed hybridization intensities the model parameters of eqn (5.15) have to be estimated in a calibration experiment. The unmethylated background intensities of all probes can be estimated by measuring unmethylated reference DNA samples[4] which gives a direct estimate for I_p^0. The dynamic range of all probes can be estimated from an additional measurement of a completely methylated reference samples.[5] It is simply the difference between methylated and unmethylated reference sample intensities $k_p = I_p^1 - I_p^0$. The methylation rate can be computed as

$$M_p = \frac{\max(I_p - I_p^0, 0)}{I_p^1 - I_p^0}, \qquad (5.16)$$

where I_p^0 and I_p^1 are the calibration measurements of probe p from the unmethylated and methylated reference samples. The maximum function is used to avoid negative methylation rates. Probes with $I_p^1 \leq I_p^0$ (or $I_p^1 \geq I_p^0$ for non-methylation probes) do not work properly and should be excluded from analysis. For bisulphite microarrays the equation splits into two independent estimators for methylation rate. The methylation detection probe gives $M_p^+ = \max(I_p^+ - I_p^{0+}, 0)/(I_p^{1+} - I_p^{0+})$ and the non-methylation detection probe gives $M_p^- = \max(I_p^{0-} - I_p^-, 0)/(I_p^{0-} - I_p^{1-})$. The two independent methylation rate estimates can be averaged to get the final methylation rate.

---

[4]Creation of unmethylated reference DNA is not trivial. One popular method is to use whole genome amplification of human DNA via phi29 polymerase. A problem with this approach is the variable copy number of different genomic locations.

[5]Completely methylated reference DNA can be generated by treating any DNA sample with SssI methylase.

A fundamental problem of the calibration method described above is that it requires the same ploidy in the used reference samples and the measured samples. This is usually not the case for CpG positions on the X and Y chromosome as well as CpG positions on aneuploid chromosomes in cancer cells. In these cases the respective methylation rate estimates will be off by a factor corresponding to the change in ploidy between reference and measurement sample. For bisulphite microarrays this issue can be avoided by using the redundant methylation and non-methylation measurements for a probe-wise calibration. In analogy to eqn (5.1) the methylation rate can be calculated as $M_p = M_p^+/(M_p^+ + M_p^-)$ and any ploidy distortions will cancel out.

If we assume that the dynamic range of methylation and non-methylation detection probes is identical the probe-wise calibrated methylation rate can be directly computed as a simple ratio of background corrected intensities:

$$M_p = \frac{\max(I_p^+ - I_p^{0+}, 0)}{\max(I_p^+ - I_p^{0+}, 0) + \max(I_p^- - I_p^{1-}, 0)}, \quad (5.17)$$

where I_p^{0+} and I_p^{1-} are unmethylated and methylated reference sample measurements. The corresponding log methylation odds are simply the log ratio of methylation and non-methylation probe intensities:

$$\log O_p = \log \frac{\max(I_p^+ - I_p^{0+}, 0)}{\max(I_p^- - I_p^{1-}, 0)}. \quad (5.18)$$

In practice the background correction is much more important than a calibration of dynamic ranges and these simplified equations give good estimates for methylation rate and log methylation odds (Adorjan et al., 2002; Bibikova et al., 2006).

5.4 Data analysis

After preprocessing DNA methylation data (e.g. represented as log methylation odds) and mRNA expression data (e.g. represented as log mRNA concentrations) show very similar distributions and correlation structures. Biological and clinical questions that have to be answered are also very similar. Therefore statistical methods established in the context of microarray or realtime PCR based expression analysis can usually be readily applied to the analysis of DNA methylation patterns. This includes methods for experimental design, hypothesis testing and correction for multiple comparisons, clustering, and classification (Speed, 2003; Draghici, 2003). In the following we will give three typical examples of methylation data analysis.

5.4.1 Tissue classification using DNA microarrays

Our first example (Model et al., 2001) consists of cell lines and primary tissue obtained from patients with acute lymphoblastic leukemia (ALL) or acute myeloid leukemia (AML). A total of 17 ALL and 8 AML samples were included.

The methylation status of these samples was evaluated at 81 CpG dinucleotide positions by using a bisulphite microarray. Measurement values are represented as log methylation odds. The analysis objective is to find an algorithm that can discriminate between ALL and AML based on the methylation pattern of a subset of the 81 analysed CpG dinucleotides.

Here we will use the support vector machine algorithm (Christianini and Shawe-Taylor, 2000) for classification. The major problem of all classification algorithms for methylation and expression microarray data analysis alike is the high dimension of input space compared to the small number of available samples. Although the support vector machine is designed to overcome this problem it still suffers from these extreme conditions. Therefore feature selection is of crucial importance for good performance (Blum and Langley, 1997) and we give special consideration to it by comparing several methods on the data set.

5.4.1.1 *Support vector machines* In our case, the task of cancer classification consists of constructing a machine that can predict the leukemia subtype (ALL or AML) from a patient's methylation pattern. For every patient sample this pattern is given as log methylation odds d_{ip}, where i is the respective patient sample index and p a specific CpG position. The complete patient methylation profile is given by the vector $\mathbf{d}_i = (d_{i1}, \ldots, d_{in_p})'$.

Based on a given set of training examples $D = \{\mathbf{d}_i : \mathbf{d}_i \in R^{n_p}\}$ with known diagnosis $Y = \{y_i : y_i \in \{\text{ALL}, \text{AML}\}\}$ a discriminant function $f : R^{n_p} \to \{\text{ALL}, \text{AML}\}$, where n_p is the number of CpG positions, has to be learned. The number of misclassifications of f on the training set $\{D, Y\}$ is called the training error and is usually minimized by the learning machine during the training phase. However, what is of practical interest is the capability to predict the class of previously unseen samples, the so-called generalization performance of the learning machine. This performance is usually estimated by the test error, which is the number of misclassifications on an independent test set $\{D', Y'\}$.

The major problem of training a learning machine with good generalization performance is to find a discriminant function f which on the one hand is complex enough to capture the essential properties of the data distribution, but which on the other hand avoids over-fitting the data. The support vector machine (SVM) tries to solve this problem by constructing a linear discriminant that separates the training data and maximizes the distance to the nearest points of the training set. This discriminant is also referred to as the maximum margin hyperplane and has very good generalization properties.

Of course there are more complex classification problems, where the dependence between class labels y_i and features $\mathbf{d}_i$ is not linear and the training set cannot be separated by a hyperplane. In order to allow for nonlinear discriminant functions the input space can be nonlinearly mapped into a potentially higher dimensional feature space by a mapping function $\Phi : \mathbf{d}_i \to \Phi(\mathbf{d}_i)$. Because the SVM algorithm in its dual formulation uses only the inner product between elements of the input space, knowledge of the kernel function

$k(\mathbf{d}_i, \mathbf{d}_j) = \langle \Phi(\mathbf{d}_i), \Phi(\mathbf{d}_j) \rangle$ is sufficient to train the SVM (Christianini and Shawe-Taylor, 2000). It is not necessary to explicitly know the mapping Φ and a nonlinear SVM can be trained efficiently by computing only the kernel function. Here we will only use the linear kernel $k(\mathbf{d}_i, \mathbf{d}_j) = \langle \mathbf{d}_i, \mathbf{d}_j \rangle$ and the quadratic kernel $k(\mathbf{d}_i, \mathbf{d}_j) = (\langle \mathbf{d}_i, \mathbf{d}_j \rangle + 1)^2$.

In the next section we will compare SVMs trained on different feature sets. In order to evaluate the prediction performance of these SVMs we used a cross-validation method (Bishop, 1995). For each classification task, the samples were partitioned into eight groups of approximately equal size. Then the SVM predicted the class for the test samples in one group after it had been trained using the seven other groups. The number of misclassifications was counted over eight runs of the SVM algorithm for all possible choices of the test group. To obtain a reliable estimate for the test error the number of misclassifications was averaged over 50 different partitionings of the samples into eight groups.

5.4.1.2 *Feature selection* The simplest way for applying a SVM to our methylation data is to use every CpG position as a separate dimension, not making any assumption about the interdependence of CpG sites from the same gene. On the leukemia subclassification task the SVM with linear kernel trained on this 81 dimensional input space had an average test error of 16%. Using a quadratic kernel did not significantly improve the results (see Table 5.1). An obvious explanation for this relatively poor performance is that we have only 25 data points (even less in the training set) in a 81 dimensional space. Finding a separating hyperplane under these conditions is a heavily under-determined problem. And as it turns out, the SVM technique of maximizing the margin is not sufficient to

TABLE 5.1. Performance of different feature selection methods.

	Training Error 2 Features	Test Error 2 Features	Training Error 5 Features	Test Error 5 Features
Linear Kernel				
Fisher Criterion	0.01	0.05	0.00	0.03
PCA	0.13	0.21	0.05	0.28
No Feature Selection[†]	0.00	0.16		
Quadratic Kernel				
Fisher Criterion	0.00	0.06	0.00	0.03
PCA	0.10	0.30	0.00	0.31
Exhaustive Search	0.00	0.06	–	–
No Feature Selection[†]	0.00	0.15		

[†] The SVM was trained on all 81 features.

find the solution with optimal generalization properties. It is necessary to reduce the dimensionality of the input space while retaining the relevant information for classification. This should be possible because it can be expected that only a minority of CpG positions has any connection with the two subtypes of leukemia.

Principal component analysis Probably the most popular method for dimension reduction is principal component analysis (PCA) (Bishop, 1995). For a given training set D, PCA constructs a set of orthogonal vectors (principal components) which correspond to the directions of maximum variance. The projection of D onto the first k principal components gives the 2-norm optimal representation of D in a k-dimensional orthogonal subspace. Because this projection does not explicitly use the class information Y, PCA is an unsupervised learning technique.

In order to reduce the dimension of the input space for the SVM we performed a PCA on the combined training and test set $\{D, D'\}$ and projected both sets on the first k principal components. This gives considerably better results than performing PCA only on the training set D and is justified by the fact that no label information is used. However, the generalization results for $k = 2$ and $k = 5$, as shown in Table 5.1, were even worse than for the SVM without feature selection. The reason for this is that PCA does not necessarily extract features that are important for the discrimination between ALL and AML. It first picks the features with the highest variance, which are in this case discriminating between cell lines and primary patient tissue (see Fig. 5.4a), i.e. subgroups that

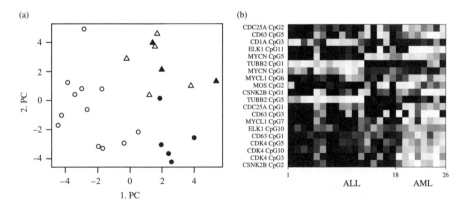

FIG. 5.4: Feature selection methods. (a) Principal component analysis. The whole data set was projected onto its first two principal components. Circles represent cell lines, triangles primary patient tissue. Filled circles or triangles are AML, empty ones ALL samples. (b) Fisher criterion. The 20 highest ranking CpG sites according to the Fisher criterion are shown. The highest ranking features are on the bottom of the plot. High probability of methylation corresponds to black, uncertainty to grey and low probability to white.

are not relevant to the classification task. Features carrying information about the leukemia subclasses appear only from the 9th principal component on. The generalization performance including the 9th component is significantly better than for a SVM without feature selection. However, it seems clear that a supervised feature selection method, which takes the class labels of the training set into account, should be more reliable and give better generalization.

Fisher criterion and t-test A classical measure to assess the degree of separation between two classes is given by the Fisher criterion (Bishop, 1995). In our case it gives the discriminative power of the kth CpG as $J(k) = (\mu_k^{ALL} - \mu_k^{AML})^2 / (\sigma_k^{ALL^2} + \sigma_k^{AML^2})$, where μ_k are the class means and σ_k are the class standard deviations. The Fisher criterion gives a high ranking for CpGs where the two classes are far apart compared to the within-class variances. Figure 5.4(b) shows the methylation profiles of the best 20 CpGs according to the Fisher criterion. Similar feature rankings can be obtained from the test statistics of univariate hypothesis tests such as the Student t-test or Wilcoxon test.

In order to improve classification performance we trained SVMs on the k highest ranking CpGs according to the Fisher criterion. The test errors for $k = 2$ and $k = 5$ are given in Table 5.1. The results show a dramatic improvement of generalization performance. Using the Fisher criterion for feature selection and $k = 5$ CpGs the test error was decreased to 3% compared to 16% for the SVM without feature selection. Analysis of the dependence of generalization performance from the selected dimension k indicates that the Fisher criterion gives dimension independent good generalization for $k < 10$.

Although the described CpG ranking methods give very good generalization, they have some potential drawbacks. One problem is that they can only detect linear dependencies between features and class labels. A simple XOR[6] or even OR[7] combination of two CpGs would be completely missed. Another drawback is that redundant features are not removed. In our case there are usually several CpGs from the same gene which have a high likelihood of comethylation. This can result in a large set of high ranking features which carry essentially the same information. Although the good results seem to indicate that the described problems do not appear in our dataset, they should be considered.

Exhaustive search PCA and Fisher criterion construct or rank features independent of the learning machine that does the actual classification and are therefore called filter methods (Blum and Langley, 1997). Another approach is to use the learning machine itself for feature selection. These techniques are called wrapper methods and try to identify the features that are important for the generalization capability of the machine. A canonical way to construct a wrapper method for feature selection is to evaluate the generalization performance of

---

[6]XOR combination: A sample is classified as positive if either CpG A or CpG B is methylated but not both.

[7]OR combination: A sample is classified as positive if either CpG A or CpG B or both are methylated.

the learning machine on every possible feature subset. Cross-validation on the training set can be used to estimate the generalization of the machine on a given feature set. What makes this exhaustive search of the feature space practically useless is the enormous number of $\sum_{k=0}^{n} \binom{n}{k} = 2^n$ different feature combinations and there are numerous heuristics to search the feature space more efficiently (e.g. backward elimination).

Here we only want to demonstrate that there are no higher order correlations between features and class labels in our data set. In order to do this we exhaustively searched the space of all two feature combinations. For each of the $\binom{81}{2} = 3240$ two CpG combinations we computed the leave-one-out cross-validation error of a SVM with quadratic kernel on the training set. From all CpG pairs with minimum leave-one-out error we selected the one with the smallest radius margin ratio.[8] This pair was considered to be the optimal feature combination and was used to evaluate the generalization performance of the SVM on the test set.

The average test error of the exhaustive search method was with 6% the same as the one of the Fisher criterion in the case of two features and a quadratic kernel. For five features the exhaustive computation is already infeasible. In the absolute majority of cross-validation runs the CpGs selected by exhaustive search and the Fisher criterion were identical. In some cases suboptimal CpGs were chosen by the exhaustive search method. These results clearly demonstrate that there are no second order combinations of two features in our data set that are important for an ALL vs. AML discrimination. We expect that higher than second order combinations of more than two features cannot be detected reliably with such a limited sample size. Therefore the Fisher criterion should be able to extract all classification relevant information from our data set and a SVM trained on these features is the optimal classifier for this application.

5.4.2 Plasma based cancer detection

Our second example (Lofton-Day et al., 2008) consists of plasma samples collected from 179 healthy individuals, and 133 patients with colorectal cancer (CRC) from the same age group. The concentration of methylated DNA in the plasma samples was measured for three different genes (TMEFF2, NGFR, SEPT9). In addition the concentration of bisulphite converted DNA was measured independent of methylation status (bisDNA). The analysis objective is to find the gene or gene combination that can most accurately discriminate between normal and CRC samples based on the measured plasma DNA concentrations.

In the following description of plasma marker analysis we will first look at the classification performance of individual marker genes. Then we will evaluate whether a combination of several genes into a marker panel can improve classification performance by using logistic regression analysis.

---

[8]The ratio between the radius of the minimum sphere enclosing all data points and the margin of the separating hyperplane.

TABLE 5.2. Single marker performance in plasma.

	TMEFF2	NGFR	SEPT9	BisDNA
Qualitative Analysis				
Normal Plasma Positives in %[†]	31 (24–38)	16 (11–23)	14 (9–20)	100
CRC Plasma Positives in %[†]	65 (56–73)	51 (42–60)	69 (60–77)	100
Quantitative Analysis				
AUC	0.72	0.70	0.80	0.61
Wilcoxon P-Value	0	0	0	0.0001
Cutoff for 95% Specificity in mg/L[*]	0.098	0.019	0.011	150.3
Sensitivity at 95% Specificity in %[*]	30	33	52	15

[†] 95% confidence intervals in parenthesis.
[*] The DNA concentration cutoff was selected to correctly classify 95% of normal samples as negative. Sensitivity gives the percentage of cancer samples that are correctly classified as positive when this cutoff is used.

5.4.2.1 *Single marker analysis* Because hypermethylation of specific genes is exclusively associated with cancer, methylation markers are typically highly specific for tumour DNA derived from cancer patients compared to normal individuals, and the simplest way to analyse them is qualitatively. This means a positive measurement value (i.e. the presence of an amplification curve) is a positive classification as *CRC*, a negative measurement value (i.e. the absence of an amplification curve) is a negative classification as *Normal*. The resulting positive rates can be directly interpreted as sensitivity (positive rate in CRC) and specificity (100% minus positive rate in Normals) and results for our example are shown in Table 5.2. For computation of confidence intervals the binomial distribution or its normal approximation can be used.

Despite their high specificity most methylation markers have a significant positive rate in normal plasma. The concentration of methylated DNA in a particular plasma sample carries therefore additional information that might improve classification by using a quantitative classification cutoff. Whether there is a significant difference in concentrations of methylated DNA between the normal and the cancer class can be assessed with a simple two-sample hypothesis test, e.g. the Wilcoxon–Mann–Whitney test. The degree of quantitative discrimination can be assessed by analysing the receiver operating characteristic (ROC) curve (Pepe, 2003). The area under the ROC curve (AUC) is a general measure for how well a marker discriminates between two classes that can be used without specifying the cost of false positives and false negatives. The ROC curves for our example are shown in Fig. 5.5(a) and corresponding AUC values are given in Table 5.2. The concrete choice of a cutoff depends on the application and

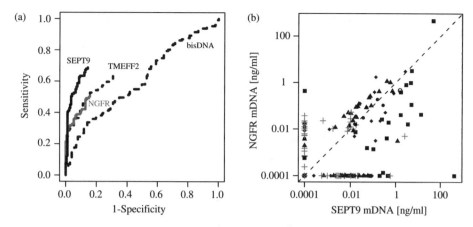

FIG. 5.5: Plasma based CRC detection. (a) Receiver operating characteristic curves of TMEFF2, NGFR, SEPT9 and total bisulphite assays for the discrimination between normal and CRC plasma. (b) Correlation between plasma concentrations of methylated DNA from SEPT9 and NGFR real-time PCR assays on a set of normal patients (grey; crosses) and patients with colorectal cancer (black; stage 0/I points, stage II diamonds, stage III triangles, stage IV squares, unknown stage open circles).

its requirements with regard to sensitivity and specificity. An application of our markers for early detection of cancer would for example require a high specificity since the prevalence of cancer in the asymptomatic population is low and even a moderate false positive rate would incur considerable costs.

5.4.2.2 *Marker panel analysis using logistic regression* In complex diseases like cancer the existence of alternative genetic mechanisms represented by complementary activation or deactivation of marker genes has to be considered. In our plasma data set the number of markers is so small that in contrast to the microarray example all possible feature combinations can be evaluated. As an alternative to the SVM algorithm of the last section we use a logistic regression model. Compared with the SVM, logistic regression has the disadvantages that it is restricted to linear discrimination functions and that it makes some assumptions about the data distribution. However, as we saw in the last section linear discriminants are often the optimal choice and distribution assumptions are minor. Compared to machine learning algorithms like the SVM, the advantage of logistic regression analysis is that it results in a complete statistical model that gives, for instance, confidence intervals and p-values for all parameter estimates.

The complete logistic regression model including DNA concentrations of the three methylation markers and the bisulphite DNA measurement is given by the logit function

$$g(\mathbf{d}_i) = \beta_0 + \beta_1 d_{i,\text{TMEFF2}} + \beta_2 d_{i,\text{NGFR}} + \beta_3 d_{i,\text{SEPT9}} + \beta_4 d_{i,\text{bisDNA}}, \quad (5.19)$$

TABLE 5.3. Marker panel performance in plasma.

Panel	Marker	Odds Ratio[†] (95% CI)	P Value	Bias-corrected AUC
TMEFF2+NGFR	TMEFF2	1.4 (1.2–1.6)	0.004	0.74
	NGFR	1.7 (1.5–2.0)	0.0003	
SEPT9+NGFR	SEPT9	2.6 (2.3–3.1)	<0.0001	0.81
	NGFR	1.4 (1.2–1.6)	0.04	
SEPT9+TMEFF2	SEPT9	2.8 (2.4–3.2)	<0.0001	0.81
	TMEFF2	1.3 (1.1–1.4)	0.05	
SEPT9+NGFR+ TMEFF2+bisDNA	SEPT9	2.6 (2,2–3.1)	<0.0001	0.79
	NGFR	1.2 (1.0–1.5)	0.3	
	TMEFF2	1.2 (1.0–1.4)	0.4	
	bisDNA	1.0 (0.8–1.3)	0.9	

[†] Odds are per 10-fold change of DNA concentration.

where $\mathbf{d}_i$ are the log DNA concentrations for sample i, β_0 is the model intercept, and β_1, β_2, β_3 and β_4 are the weights for methylation markers and bisulphite DNA. The probability of a patient i having cancer is then $P(y_i = CRC|\mathbf{d}_i) = e^{g(\mathbf{d}_i)}/(1 + e^{g(\mathbf{d}_i)})$. Partial models for feature subsets are simply constructed by setting the weights for the deselected features to $\beta = 0$.

Results for the complete model and all partial methylation marker models are shown in Table 5.3. Weights are given as odds ratios e^β with corresponding confidence intervals and p-values based on the Wald statistic. In addition the predictive performance of each logistic regression model is quantified with an AUC value. Since multivariate models are prone to over-fitting cross-validation has to be used for unbiased AUC estimation. Here the over-fitting bias corrected AUC values were calculated from the bootstrap corrected concordance index (C index) (Harrel, 2001). Results show that the best performing marker panel is the combination of SEPT9 and NGFR with a small but significant bias corrected AUC improvement of 1% over SEPT9 alone. Complementarity is low because the tested methylation markers are highly correlated on a subset of CRC patient samples with high tumour DNA concentrations in plasma (Fig. 5.5(b)). This analysis indicates that the single marker, SEPT9, is the best choice for a plasma based colorectal cancer detection test.

5.4.3 Cancer recurrence prediction

Our third example (Nimmrich et al., 2008) is a cohort of 412 lymph-node negative, steroid hormone receptor positive breast cancer patients who had not received any adjuvant systemic treatment. The DNA methylation rate of the PITX2 gene was measured in primary tumour tissue. After surgery all patients were examined at least twice yearly during the first 5 years of follow-up and once yearly thereafter. The median follow-up period of patients still alive at time of analysis was 98 months, 92 patients (22%) developed distant metastasis during follow-up. The analysis objective is to find out whether methylation of the PITX2 gene can predict the risk of cancer recurrence.

The distinctive property of survival analysis is the handling of incomplete follow-up observations. When a patient cohort is followed it is usually impossible to observe the end point (here cancer recurrence, i.e. development of a distant metastasis) for every patient. Many patients will have a limited follow-up time without reaching the end point – these observations are *censored*. When making predictions about patient survival the information from these censored observations has to be taken into account.

The simplest method for estimating survival probabilities is Kaplan–Meier analysis (Lawless, 2002). It computes the survival probability at a given time point as a product estimate from all earlier observations. For each observed end point the number of patients that were actually still at risk at that time is taken into account. Kaplan–Meier analysis is a univariate non-parametric method with minimal assumptions (independence between censoring and survival times).

In order to apply Kaplan–Meier analysis to our data set we have to define a PITX2 methylation cutoff that splits our sample into patient groups with potentially different prognosis. Depending on the medical expectations with regard to proportions of high and low risk groups the cutoff is usually defined as a quantile of the methylation measurement distribution. Here we define the cutoff as the 66% quantile and the resulting survival curves are shown in Fig. 5.6.

Kaplan–Meier analysis is only descriptive. In order to determine whether the observed difference between the two curves is significant we can use the

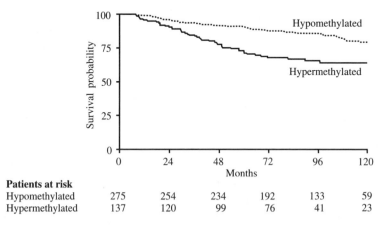

FIG. 5.6: Kaplan–Meier survival curves. Patients were split at the 66% quantile of PITX2 DNA methylation rates. The dotted line shows the estimated survival curve for the hypomethylated patient group; the solid line shows the hypermethylated patient group.

non-parametric log rank test that compares the survival distributions of two sample sets. In our case the survival distributions of the PITX2 hypo- and hypermethylated patient groups show a significant difference with $P < 0.01$.

To find out whether PITX2 methylation really is a novel and independent prognostic factor it has to be analysed in a multivariate statistical model together with established prognostic factors like age, tumour size and grade, and steroid hormone receptor levels. A Cox regression model is one way to achieve this. Details of this more advanced analysis can be found in the original article (Nimmrich et al., 2008).

5.5 Conclusions

DNA methylation plays a central role in carcinogenesis and has many promising applications, especially in cancer diagnostics. A variety of methylation measurement technologies exist and the right preprocessing algorithms for translating raw measurement signals into quantitative methylation estimates are key for obtaining accurate results. Here we have taken a closer look at preprocessing algorithms for direct bisulphite sequencing and DNA methylation microarrays. For both cases the described algorithms allow the quantification of methylation rates at single CpG resolution.

The interpretation and analysis of DNA methylation data is very similar to mRNA expression analysis. We have given three typical examples. In the case of the DNA microarray analysis example we have shown that simple univariate ranking methods like the Fisher criterion are able to select all DNA methylation features that are relevant for a given classification task. Together with a classification algorithm such as the SVM it is possible to accurately discriminate different cancer types based on their methylation patterns. The second example showed that free floating cancer DNA can be detected in the blood stream and that qualitative or quantitative analysis of a single methylation marker can discriminate between cancer patients and healthy individuals with high accuracy. The last example demonstrated how the methylation rate in tumour samples can be used to predict the probability of tumour recurrence by using simple Kaplan–Meier analysis. These examples prove that DNA methylation analysis is a powerful tool for all areas of cancer research and diagnostics.

References

Adorjan, P., Distler, J., Lipscher, E., Model, F., Muller, J., Pelet, C., Braun, A., Florl, A.R., Gutig, D., Grabs, G., Howe, A., Kursar, M., Lesche, R., Leu, E., Lewin, A., Maier, S., Muller, V., Otto, T., Scholz, C., Schulz, W.A., Seifert, H.H., Schwope, I., Ziebarth, H., Berlin, K., Piepenbrock, C., and Olek, A. (2002). Tumour class prediction and discovery by microarray-based dna methylation analysis. *Nucleic Acids Research*, **30**(5), e21.

Barton, G.J. (1993). An efficient algorithm to locate all locally optimal alignments between two sequences allowing for gaps. *Computer Applications in the Biosciences*, **9**(6), 729–34.

Bibikova, M., Lin, Z., Zhou, L., Chudin, E., Garcia, E.W., Wu, B., Doucet, D., Thomas, N.J., Wang, Y., Vollmer, E., Goldmann, T., Seifart, C., Jiang, W., Barker, D.L., Chee, M.S., Floros, J., and Fan, J.B. (2006). High-throughput DNA methylation profiling using universal bead arrays. *Genome Research*, **16**(3), 383–93.

Bishop, C.M. (1995). *Neural Networks for Pattern Recognition*. Oxford University Press, New York.

Blum, A. and Langley, P. (1997). Selection of relevant features and examples in machine learning. *Artificial Intelligence*, **97**, 245–271.

Christianini, N. and Shawe-Taylor, J. (2000). *An Introduction to Support Vector Machines*. Cambridge University Press, Cambridge.

Cottrell, S.E., Distler, J., Goodman, N.S., Mooney, S.H., Kluth, A., Olek, A., Schwope, I., Tetzner, R., Ziebarth, H., and Berlin, K. (2004). A real-time PCR assay for DNA-methylation using methylation-specific blockers. *Nucleic Acids Research*, **32**(1), e10.

Cui, H., Cruz-Correa, M., Giardiello, F.M., Hutcheon, D.F., Kafonek, D.R., Brandenburg, S., Wu, Y., He, X., Powe, N.R., and Feinberg, A.P. (2003). Loss of IGF2 imprinting: a potential marker of colorectal cancer risk. *Science*, **299**(5613), 1753–5.

Dear, S. and Staden, R. (1992). A standard file format for data from dna sequencing instruments. *DNA Sequence*, **3**(2), 107–10.

Draghici, S. (2003). *Data Analysis Tools for DNA Microarrays*. Chapman & Hall.

Eads, C.A., Danenberg, K.D., Kawakami, K., Saltz, L.B., Blake, C., Shibata, D., Danenberg, P.V., and Laird, P.W. (2000). MethyLight: a high-throughput assay to measure DNA methylation. *Nucleic Acids Research*, **28**(8), E32.

Eckhardt, F., Lewin, J., Cortese, R., Rakyan, V.K., Attwood, J., Burger, M., Burton, J., Cox, T.V., Davies, R., Down, T.A., Haefliger, C., Horton, R., Howe, K., Jackson, D.K., Kunde, J., Koenig, C., Liddle, J., Niblett, D., Otto, T., Pettett, R., Seemann, S., Thompson, C., West, T., Rogers, J., Olek, A., Berlin, K., and Beck, S. (2006). DNA methylation profiling of human chromosomes 6, 20 and 22. *Nature Genetics*, **38**(12), 1378–85. Comparative Study.

Egger, G., Liang, G., Aparicio, A., and Jones, P.A. (2004). Epigenetics in human disease and prospects for epigenetic therapy. *Nature*, **429**(6990), 457–63.

Ehrlich, M. (2003). Expression of various genes is controlled by DNA methylation during mammalian development. *Journal of Cellular Biochemistry*, **88**(5), 899–910.

Fraga, M.F. and Esteller, M. (2002). DNA methylation: a profile of methods and applications. *Biotechniques*, **33**(3), 632, 634, 636–49.

Frommer, M., McDonald, L.E., Millar, D.S., Collis, C.M., Watt, F., Grigg, G.W., Molloy, P.L., and Paul, C.L. (1992). A genomic sequencing protocol that yields a positive display of 5-methylcytosine residues in individual dna strands. *The Proceedings of the National Academy of Sciences USA*, **89**, 1827–1831.

Grady, W.M., Willis, J., Guilford, P.J., Dunbier, A.K., Toro, T.T., Lynch, H., Wiesner, G., Ferguson, K., Eng, C., Park, J.G., Kim, S.J., and Markowitz, S. (2000). Methylation of the CDH1 promoter as the second genetic hit in hereditary diffuse gastric cancer. *Nature Genetics*, **26**(1), 16–7.

Harrel, F.E. (2001). *Regression Modeling Strategies*. Springer-Verlag, New York.

Hendrich, B. and Tweedie, S. (2003). The methyl-CpG binding domain and the evolving role of DNA methylation in animals. *Trends in Genetics*, **19**(5), 269–77.

Jones, P.A. and Baylin, S.B. (2002). The fundamental role of epigenetic events in cancer. *Nature Reviews Genetics*, **3**(6), 415–28.

Laird, P.W. (2003). The power and the promise of DNA methylation markers. *Nature Reviews Cancer*, **3**(4), 253–66.

Lawless, J.F. (2002). *Statistical Models and Methods for Lifetime Data*. John Wiley, New York.

Lewin, J., Plum, A., Hildmann, T., Rujan, T., Eckhardt, F., Liebenberg, V., Lofton-Day, C., and Wasserkort, R. (2007). Comparative DNA methylation analysis in normal and tumour tissues and in cancer cell lines using differential methylation hybridisation. *The International Journal of Biochemistry and Cell Biology*, **39**(7-8), 1539–50.

Lewin, J., Schmitt, A.O., Adorjan, P., Hildmann, T., and Piepenbrock, C. (2004). Quantitative DNA methylation analysis based on four-dye trace data from direct sequencing of PCR amplificates. *Bioinformatics*, **20**(17), 3005–12.

Lofton-Day, C., Model, F., DeVos, T., Tetzner, R., Distler, J., Schuster, M., Song, X., Lesche, R., Liebenberg, V., Ebert, M., Molnar, B., Grutzmann, R., Pilarsky, C., and Sledziewski, A. (2008). DNA methylation biomarkers for blood-based colorectal cancer screening. *Clinical Chemistry*, **54**(2), 414–23.

Model, F., Adorján, P., Olek, A., and Piepenbrok, C. (2001). Feature selection for DNA methylation based cancer classification. *Bioinformatics*, **17**(1), S157–S164.

Nimmrich, I., Sieuwerts, A.M., Meijer-van Gelder, M.E., Schwope, I., Bolt-de Vries, J., Harbeck, N., Koenig, T., Hartmann, O., Kluth, A., Dietrich, D., Magdolen, V., Portengen, H., Look, M.P., Klijn, J.G., Lesche, R., Schmitt, M., Maier, S., Foekens, J.A., and Martens, J.W. (2008). DNA hypermethylation of PITX2 is a marker of poor prognosis in untreated lymph node-negative hormone receptor-positive breast cancer patients. *Breast Cancer Research and Treatment*. **111**(3), 429–37, Epub 2007 Oct 28.

Pepe, M.S. (2003). *The Statistical Evaluation of Medical Tests for Classification and Prediction*. Oxford University Press.

Speed, T. (ed.) (2003). *Statistical Analysis of Gene Expression Microarray Data*. Chapman & Hall.

Stekel, D. (2003). *Microarray Bioinformatics*. Cambridge University Press, Cambridge.

Weber, M., Davies, J.J., Wittig, D., Oakeley, E.J., Haase, M., Lam, W.L., and Schubeler, D. (2005). Chromosome-wide and promoter-specific analyses identify sites of differential DNA methylation in normal and transformed human cells. *Nature Genetics*, **37**(8), 853–62.

Yan, P.S., Perry, M.R., Laux, D.E., Asare, A.L., Caldwell, C.W., and Huang, T.H. (2000). CpG island arrays: an application toward deciphering epigenetic signatures of breast cancer. *Clinical Cancer Research*, **6**(4), 1432–8.

6

PATHWAY ANALYSIS: PATHWAY SIGNATURES AND CLASSIFICATION

Ming Yi and Robert M. Stephens

Although the use of DNA microarrays and other high throughput (HTP) technologies is increasingly widespread and affordable, retrieval and interpretation of underlying biological themes from HTP data remains a major challenge in the area of systems biology. In recent years, pathway analysis has emerged as a category of promising analysis methods for HTP data, which is getting more and more attention in genomics and other 'omics' fields in both academic and industrial settings. This chapter focuses specifically on pathway-based analysis of HTP data. First, we provide a brief overview of pathway analysis concepts and methodologies. Then, we describe the evolution from gene signatures to pathway signatures focusing on the recent development of applications of pathways to the classification of a phenotype of interest using HTP data.

6.1 Overview of pathway analysis

6.1.1 *Pathway and network visualization methods*

Pathways have been used for graphically displaying and interpreting biological processes in biomedical research for a long time. Since the Human Genome Project gave a genome-scale view to biologists, a picture of an active cell or organism could be envisioned as an interconnected information network, with molecular components linked to one another in topologies that can encode and represent many features of biological processes and cellular function. This networked view of biology along with pathway-level details brings the potential for systematic understanding of molecular systems of living entities.

Probably the earliest pathway visualization web interface was built by the Kyoto Encyclopedia of Genes and Genomes (KEGG) group (Nakao et al., 1999). Subsequently, it was improved to have limited capacity to display microarray data within the context of pathways annotated in the KEGG pathways database (Kanehisa et al., 2002). Additional signal transduction pathways can also be visualized through the BioCarta pathway collections web site (www.biocarta.com/genes/allpathways.asp) and the Science STKE Cell Signaling pathway database web site (http://stke.sciencemag.org/cm/), although these sites were designed primarily for capture, curation, and sharing of the actual pathway data and do not allow visualization of HTP data in the context of the pathways. Until recently, software tools were implemented to incorporate pathway contents mainly for the purpose of visualizing and analysing high-throughput data. These tools include GenMAPP (Dahlquist et al., 2002), Pathway Processor (Grosu et al., 2002), and Pathway Tool (Karp et al., 2002). Thereafter, numerous pathway visualization tools were developed to provide a variety of functionalities that attempt to interpret the data within the context of pathways or directly visualize the data within pathways with colour cues. Examples of tools include but are not limited to Cytoscape (Shannon et al., 2003), ViMac (Luyf et al., 2002), Osprey (Breitkreutz et al., 2003), WPS (Yi et al., 2006), and PathSys (Baitaluk et al., 2006).

Many of these tools have one or more unique features that distinguish it from the others. Among them, it should be noted that Cytoscape (Shannon et al., 2003) has become more and more utilized since its creation. One reason is likely because Cytoscape has been evolving into a very powerful and flexible tool with many nice features, many of which are provided by plug-in packages contributed by collaborators (www.cytoscape.org/). This is probably due to two factors: plug-ins as functional extensions can be developed by anyone using the Cytoscape open Java software architecture, and public contribution has been encouraged (www.cytoscape.org/). In addition, its success and popularity have been stimulated by the Cytoscape forum, which has been extended by use from the Institute of Systems Biology and many other collaborators (http://www.cytoscape.org/). The increase in Cytoscape's popularity and success reaffirms the notion that the modular and open software implementations are highly desirable to the community.

Most of the pathway analysis tools focus more on visualization of data in the context of pathways, and only some tools may provide statistical assessment of the reliability of each differentially expressed gene (Grosu et al., 2002). Some of them tend to be comprehensive tools in addition to providing unique features. For example, WPS attempts to be a comprehensive tool with many utility functions in addition to its unique way of data visualization of pathways and networks (Yi et al., 2006). WPS is probably the first pathway analysis tool that allows simultaneous visualization of multiple HTP data in the context of one or multiple pathways and provides colour cue-based pattern extraction for genes with certain defined patterns (Yi et al., 2006). WPS is also probably the first tool that attempted to integrate analysis results from enrichment analysis or over-representation analysis with networks of genes and associated pathways or terms.

Over the years, commercial software packages including Pathway Studio (Nikitin et al., 2003; a product of Ariadne Genomics, www.ariadnegenomics.com), PathArt (a product of Jubilant Biosys Ltd, www.jubilantbiosys.com), Ingenuity Pathways Analysis tool (a product of Ingenuity Systems Inc, www.ingenuity.com/), MetaCore (a product of GeneGO Inc, www.genego.com), and Genomatix software suite GmbH (a product of Genomatix, www.genomatix.de) also joined the competition in the field of pathway-based HTP data analysis. These tools provided a variety of interfaces for the visualization of gene networks extracted by natural language processing (NLP), or hand-curated biological pathway/association networks from literature mining, and usually accepted genelist based data input for data integration. Some of the tools have nice integration with enrichment analysis and promoter analysis such as the Genomatix promoter analysis module MatInspector (Cartharius et al., 2005) and BiblioSphere module (Scherf et al., 2005) as well as the Ingenuity Pathway tool. Although industrial development teams gave these tools the advantage of cutting-edge software development technology and database capacity, including hand-curated data from literature sources, they still do not appear to be superior to what the collective academic counterparts can offer, particularly considering the expensive license fees of the industry tools compared to free availability of academic tools. Of course, the ultimate tool selected will need to weigh cost against utility and other factors.

The general usage of these tools usually begins with identifying differentially expressed genes using statistical methods, such as Significance Analysis of Microarray (Tusher et al., 2001), moderated t-test (Smyth 2005, Smyth et al., 2003), Local-Pooled-Error (LPE) (Jain et al., 2003), False Discovery Rate (FDR) (Storey and Tibshirani, 2003), as well as other gene selection methods. The latter includes the 'unusual ratio method' (Tao et al., 1999), analysis of variance (ANOVA) related methods (Draghici et al., 2001, Draghici et al., 2003; Nadon and Shoemaker 2002; Pavlidis et al., 2002; Pavlidis, 2003), and Mixed Model Analysis (Hsieh et al., 2003; Chu et al., 2002), colour cue-based pattern extraction methods (Yi et al., 2006) and patterned genes using clustering analysis; e.g. hierarchical (Eisen et al., 1998), K-means (Hartigan And Wong 1979), and Self-Organizing Maps (SOM) (Tamayo et al., 1999). Typically, these gene lists are generated outside of the pathway analysis tools using additional software tools. There are some pathway analysis tools that allow direct usage of whole data sets for analysis instead of gene lists; e.g. GenMAPP (Dahlquist et al., 2002) and WPS (Yi et al., 2006). These tools allow inclusion of all possible parameters in the data sets to set up colour cues for the visualization of data on a backdrop of pathways.

The next step typically is to use the pathway/network-based tools to map the critical genes into the context of pathways or biological networks and seek the connection of these genes within pathways and networks for clues of embedded biological themes by means of colour cues for data integration, gene-gene or gene-term association relations implicated by connections of nodes in pathways or networks, and higher levels of network features such as hubs derived from graphical layout of network architecture. Some tools have the capacity to use the results of enrichment analysis to filter and simplify the networks to focus on specific subdomains of the networks or subnetworks; these tools include WPS (Yi et al., 2006). Others such as Cytoscape (Shannon et al., 2003), MintViewer (Zanzoni et al., 2002), and Osprey (Breitkreutz et al., 2003) focusing more on network views and queries of the data, have included features for viewing and querying larger subsets of the networks of association relations such as the interactome on a more global scale. These tools typically operate from the viewpoint of physical associations between proteins, or correlated gene expression, and include information that summarizes annotated functions, such as Gene Ontology (GO), groupings among subnetworks of linked genes or proteins. One tool named VisANT (Hu et al., 2004), which attempts to integrate interactome data from different sources, has the ability to uncover orthologous networks, and perform exploratory data mining and basic graph operations on arbitrary networks and subnetworks, including loop detection, degree distribution (the distribution of edges per node) and shortest path identification between various component (genes or proteins). Commercial counterparts such as the Ingenuity Pathway tool (www.ingenuity.com), MetaCore of GeneGo (www.genego.com) can do similar operations and queries as well. Some very recent efforts have focused more on exploring the topology and architectures of the networks in conjunction with high-throughput data to seek biological scenarios (Lu et al., 2007; Ulitsky and Shamir 2007).

Each of the existing tools shows strengths and weaknesses in addition to all of their unique capabilities. The differences typically fall into two categories. In the first category, there are differences in data visualization capabilities. This reflects the tools' ability to lay out the pathway or network and allow the user to interact with it. These tools also include methods whereby the data provided by the user is overlaid onto the pathways. Some tools have a cumbersome interface requiring the user to switch between different experiments and remember what the other screens looked like. A second class of tool variation comes from the source or sources of pathway data. Pathway data can be derived from natural language processing, which is error prone but relatively exhaustive compared to some other pathway derivation methods. The opposite extreme is to hand curate the data by expert reading of the literature to build a set of pathways derived from experimentally identified physical or genetic interaction data. Yet another source of pathway information can be derived from other terms, such as GO terms where groups of genes sharing a particular functional term can be grouped together into a hypothetical pathway or group. Similarly, other groupings through transcription factor binding sites, miRNA target interactions, etc., can also be useful. Together, this again encourages a relatively modular approach to software design whereby different visualization views can be combined with different pathways to provide the ultimate in flexibility.

Given the variety of pathway and network analysis tools available for the community, pathway information and related databases covering not just traditional metabolic or signalling pathways, but also relevant information such as protein–protein interaction, genetic interaction, gene regulation, or transcriptional regulation, have greatly expanded over the years (Cary et al., 2005). A pathway modelling language is critically needed that can best capture and exchange with other systems the pathway information derived from a diversity of pathway databases with enormously different data models, data access methods, file formats and semantic differences in different data sources. Some efforts to accomplish this have been made, such as Systems Biology Markup Language (SBML) (Hucka et al., 2003) and its derivatives including PSI-MI/ CellML (Lloyd et al., 2004) and BioPAX (www.biopax.org).

It should be pointed out that due to the relatively large number of network and pathway tools available for biologists and bioinformaticians, the decision of which tool should be used for each application can be a complex process that often involves personal preferences as much as anything else. Side-by-side comparisons among the tools should be made to help users make the best use of the tools. Some comparative efforts have been made (Suderman et al., 2007; Yi et al., 2006), but more extensive efforts using global and systematic comparisons would be really helpful for different levels of users that have different analysis goals in mind: e.g. an unbiased complete survey of the uniqueness and advantages of each of these tools would be welcome. Ranking these tools in different important aspects of their applications to address these issues would also be useful, although such a task appears to be really difficult and may have concerns about objectivity. Such a comparison task is further complicated by the fact that many of the applications are considered 'works in progress' with additional features and capabilities being added almost daily.

6.1.2 Gene-set based methods

In addition to pathway/network based analysis approaches, there is a category of related but different methods based upon pre-declared gene sets. A gene set is a collection of genes that have some functional relevance or relationship and were put together as a group or a set, which were annotated or represented for a certain biological meaning; e.g. GO terms, or Gene Set Enrichment Analysis (GSEA) annotation terms. In the broader pathway definition, a pathway consists of not only a set of genes, but also includes some physical connection or gene-to-gene relations, usually presented graphically. This conceptual 'pathway' consists of a set of genes that are physically grouped or linked together as a functional unit to perform a well-known biological function or constitute a defined biological process (e.g. KEGG pathways: www.genome.jp/kegg/; Biocarta pathways: www.biocarta.com/genes/allpathways.asp). In contrast to a pathway-based method, a gene-set based approach only considers the fact that the genes in a defined gene set are grouped together based on their association with an annotation term or common functional or structural feature, but without regard to information of any direct relationship such as protein–protein interaction, kinase vs. substrate, etc.

Gene-set based analysis methods, also referred to as modular methods, include but are not restrict to enrichment-based analysis (or over-representation analysis), functional class scoring (FCS), global tests, and singular value decomposition (SVD) methods.

Over-representation analysis (ORA), sometimes called enrichment analysis, begins with pre-defined gene lists (e.g. differential genes between tumour and normal tissues), which are subjected to analysis for enrichment levels that evaluate which functional categories are represented in the lists more than expected by chance. These methods are usually based on a one-tailed Fisher's exact test or similarly derived enrichment scores (Hosack et al., 2003; Al-Shahrour et al., 2004; Yi et al., 2006). ORA has been widely used to seek biological themes embedded or represented by gene lists that are differentially expressed with certain functional or structural features. Many software tools have implemented this algorithm including but not limited to EASE/DAVID (Hosack et al., 2003; Dennis et al., 2003), GOminer (Zeeberg et al., 2003); Fatigo (Al-Shahrour et al., 2004), T-profiler (Boorsma et al., 2005), and WPS (Yi et al., 2006). One caveat for such methods is that since they present a ranked list of terms based on the Fisher's exact test p-values or enrichment type of scores, they are quite sensitive to the cutoff value used for getting the gene lists (Pavlidis et al., 2004).

In contrast, functional class scoring (FCS) usually starts with all genes from a data set ranked based on their expression differences in terms of statistical significance (e.g., t-test p-values between the two classes and p-value based aggregate scoring FCS method (Pavlidis et al., 2004)), based on their expression differences in terms of fold change versus a normal distribution (Kim and Volsky, 2005), based on correlation levels between their expression in the two classes (e.g. the signal to noise ratio (SNR) in GSEA method (Mootha et al., 2003, Subramanian et al., 2005, Sweet-Cordero et al., 2005)), or based on correlated expression patterns (Lamb et al., 2003). Once these rankings, statistical values, or correlation levels of individual genes are derived, aggregate class scores for functional categories are derived with different algorithms that rank the functional terms. The most popular one in this category is probably the GSEA method (www.broad.mit.edu/gsea/). The GSEA method has recently been improved by the addition of more GSEA annotation terms as well as the ability to deal with terms or gene sets of different sizes (Mootha et al., 2003; Subramanian et al., 2005), since it was argued by others that the GSEA method may be biased toward assigning higher enrichment scores to gene sets of large size (Damian and Gorfine, 2004).

Other related methods include the global test method, which looks for associations between the global expression pattern for a group of genes and a variable of interest (e.g. a clinical outcome) (Goeman et al., 2004). A SVD method has been developed that uses the first metagene derived from singular value decomposition as the basis for calculation of a defined pathway activity level (Tomfohr et al., 2005).

It should be emphasized that the common gene-level statistical approaches have encountered limitations when no individual genes meet the threshold for statistical significance (Mootha et al., 2003), because the relevant biological differences are modest compared to the noise inherent in microarray technology or biological variations across individual samples (e.g. genetic background). As mentioned above, one popular FCS analysis method, namely GSEA, has been developed to overcome such limitations by combining the power of ranking of individual genes for functional class scoring (Mootha et al., 2003; Subramanian et al., 2005). The method has been further extended to incorporate cross-species gene expression analysis as a new strategy of using genomic analysis from animal models to probe human diseases (Sweet-Cordero et al., 2005).

6.2 From gene signatures/classifiers to pathway signatures/classifiers

6.2.1 Gene signature and classifiers

Gene signatures have usually been referred to as sets of genes whose change in behaviour (e.g. transcription level, protein expression levels) reflect the change of biological states or stages of disease progression. Some of the gene signatures have been used as biomarkers or therapeutical targets. Usually, signature genes were identified and then confirmed in follow-up studies. In other cases, signature genes have been used to develop classifiers or predictive models for the purpose of class prediction.

Most, if not all, conventional gene-level paradigm-based methods start with a single list of differentially expressed genes based on the assumption that, for a given phenotype (e.g. tumour vs. normal tissues, treated vs. control), any relevant genes should behave consistently across the samples or individuals within the studied population and class (e.g. tumour or normal tissues). In other words, they generally focus on evaluating and selecting genes with statistically significant changes in expression patterns at the individual gene level across the entire data set. Such selection methods are either based on fold change or altered ratios as evaluated by t-test derived statistical methods that consider the mean values of the two classes (e.g. tumour vs. normal), p-values, and FDRs. Other methods are based on more complex models including ANOVA (Nadon et al., 2002; Kerr et al., 2000, Pavlidis et al., 2003), ANOVA-based noise sampling method (Draghici et al., 2001, 2003b), and mixed-model analysis (MMA method, Hsieh et al., 2003; Chu et al., 2002) that consider complex variance analysis or contributions to the abundance of variance among individuals and between the contrasted classes, as well as estimation of empirical distribution of noise with replicate spots. These methods tend to summarize the statistical differences for each gene between two classes into a single parametric value. Such gene-level paradigm-based methods tend to derive a single list of genes summarized from the analysis for the intended class comparison, which reflects how well the changes of each gene across samples correlate with phenotype. The methods have been successfully used to identify many critical gene signatures and biomarkers that persistently exist within the sample population or are associated with phenotypic changes.

Such gene-level paradigm-based gene selection methods usually use metrics that are computed across samples from the two classes and require inter-sample consistencies within a class. Several inadequacies for these selection methods have been encountered where genes with large variances in the sample population have a better chance of exhibiting unrealistically large fold changes, even if they are not differentially expressed. Similarly, genes with only a small fold change may have a very small p-value because of a very small standard deviation. Even the suggestion by the MicroArray Quality Control consortium that fold change ranking plus a non-stringent p-value cutoff can be used as a baseline for generating more reproducible signature gene lists (MAQC Consortium 2006) has been questioned (Perket, 2006). Thus, it appears that signature genes for a given system are affected by the choice of algorithm or statistical method that is chosen to derive these signatures, given the intention of signatures to represent the distinct features of studied system at the gene level.

This is similarly true for gene signatures derived for the purpose of classifiers in many classification or class prediction methods. Class prediction is a supervised learning method where the algorithm learns from a training set (known samples) and establishes a prediction rule or model to classify new samples. When microarray data were just starting to be used for more and more biological studies, they were quickly tested and used for classification of phenotypes or diseases including different cancer types and subtypes (Golub et al., 1999). There are numerous well-known classification methods, including but not limited to Random Forest (Breiman et al., 2001), Support Vector Machine (Vapnik 1995; Guyon et al., 2002), Thrunken Centroids or PAM (Tibshirani et al., 2002), and Diagonal Linear Discriminant Analysis (DLDA) (Dudoit et al., 2002). Many classification methods select genes based on their ranking according to their predictive accuracy (discriminatory ability for the contrasted classes) with a procedure of gene-by-gene prediction and the frequency of selections in cross-validation (Li et al., 2001; Guyon et al., 2002; Cho et al., 2004). Some recent efforts for gene selection have used multiple layers of ranking algorithms for gene ranking with different criteria, where each individual criterion has a separate contribution to its ordering of preference for selection (Chen et al., 2007). Other recent methods included CERP, which is based on the Classification and Regression Tree (CART) algorithm (Moon et al., 2006). More comprehensive gene signatures have been derived using integrative analysis methods including the meta-analysis method (Rhodes and Chinnaiyan 2005), which has been developed to derive different robust gene signatures that can characterize myriad subtypes of a variety of cancers.

Although the potential benefit to the application of these signatures is obvious, one important issue regarding the identification and use of the classifiers is the overfitting problem. In particular, the overfitting problem exists for many methods that have greater propensity to capitalize on chance, or 'overfit' the sample data on which the model is derived (Tibshirani, 1996). In typical HTP experiments with thousands or even millions of data points and typically low numbers of experiments (10s–100s), it is quite easy to identify lists of random features that could function as classifiers. The goal of model building for classifiers is to obtain a predictive model that generalizes across many such samples to the universe at large, and not merely to the samples at hand. The consequence of overfitting is that individual models will overfit their training data and not generalize well to other data. Thus, small changes in training data can have considerable influence on the outcome of the learning exercise and models will have high variance. Increasing the sample size, which could address the overfitting problem in theory, is not always feasible or even effective (Dobbin and Simon, 2007). Alternatively, cross-validation can largely prevent or reduce the risk of overfitting. However, there might still be an issue if a substantial amount of non-sampling errors (e.g. due to different technological devices) are present (Ntzani and Loannidis, 2003; Michiels et al., 2005). Thus, testing the classifiers across different experimental systems remains an extremely important component to the elucidation and validation of the classifier gene signatures. Since pathways or gene sets are collections of genes of assumed or validated functional relationships, making explanatory or predictive models at the level of pathways or gene sets may simplify the models that previously relied on genes. Such pathway-level classifiers may possibly be less susceptible to the overfitting problem due to aggregation of gene-level variables, although costs may be associated with the modelling processes when going from genes to pathways. Thus, pathway classifiers for predictive models or pathway signatures for explanatory models may tend to be more reliable than their gene-based counterparts.

6.2.2 Pathway signatures/classifiers as an alternative?

Given the 'vulnerability' of gene signatures and gene classifiers in terms of the influence that choice of method and algorithm have upon their content, biologists probably would prefer to see more reliable signatures of changes or distinct biological differences that characterize a specific biological system under study regardless of the measuring method or analysis algorithm and method that has been used to derive such signatures. The inherent complexity of biological systems, the multiple stages where protein function can be regulated and the high overall levels of individual variation suggest that gene-level signatures or gene-level classification-based approaches may miss important aspects of biology due to their susceptibility to the choice of algorithm or methodology. For example, many complex diseases, including cancers, heart disease, and hypertension, are not simply caused by a single gene, but have been shown to be caused by mutations in multiple genes in the same or related pathways (Peltonen et al., 2001; Scott et al., 2001; Reiter et al., 2001; Dohr et al., 2005). In addition, the gene-by-gene approach or gene-level paradigm fails to put single genes in an overall functional context, and consequently ignores other relevant genes that have biological relevance and also show similar expression profiles or correlation with the phenotypes under study.

Evidence has shown that many pathway/gene-set based analysis methods or group testing methods identify the same pathways that had already been shown to be involved in the pathogenesis of prostate cancer derived from different prostate data sets, and these pathways/gene-sets appeared to be more consistent than simple gene signatures (Manoli et al., 2006). Moreover, pathways recurrently identified in these analyses are more likely to be reliable than those from a single analysis on a single data set (Manoli et al., 2006). While biologically relevant genes may consistently behave in correlation with an associated phenotype across a population, it is even more likely that common pathways can be impacted through distinct gene events that are not reflected at the individual gene level. This seems particularly relevant considering the stochastic nature of many epigenetic events that lead to disease states. These and similar observations have driven the efforts to evolve the gene-level signatures to pathway-level or gene-set-level signatures, or from gene-based classification methods to pathway or gene-set-based classification methods. The pathway-based signatures seem likely to evolve further as the interconnectivity and details of known and to-be-identified pathways emerge through various technologies that are now being applied.

There are several reasons why a pathway-level, gene-set-based, or modular analysis scheme may be superior to conventional methods that rely on a gene-level paradigm-based analysis scheme. First, external stimuli that lead to the same phenotypic responses may not necessarily cause the same specific regulatory changes in different individuals. Instead, for each individual case, different genes at different steps of the same biological process that leads to the phenotype or response may actually be involved. For example, inappropriate expression of a ligand or expression of a ligand-independent form of a receptor can invoke the same effect. Secondly, as mentioned above, more complex diseases such as cancers, Parkinson's disease, and hypertension may involve multiple processes and multiple genes. In individuals with such complex diseases, the genetic alternations may occur through different genes instead of a single gene. Even for the same genes, the changes may occur at the level of protein expression, transcription, post-translational modifications, and/or signaling/metabolic products. Thirdly, most current high-throughput approaches, including microarrays measuring the transcriptome, mass spectroscopy or other proteomic HTP measurements for the proteome, metabolic profiling for the metabolome, and electron transfer dissociation (ETD) for phosphorylation or phosphopeptides, each only measures one level of changes. Each of the methods mentioned above only generates data regarding one aspect of the changes across the genes and can only discover the genes or proteins with changes at one level on their own data set. With conventional gene-level analysis methods, genes have to be uniformly changed at one level (e.g. transcription level, or protein expression level) consistently across the sample class populations in order to be included into the 'differentiated' or 'significantly' changed list.

No gene operates in a vacuum: each gene interacts either directly or indirectly through its protein product with many other genes and gene products (Peltonen *et al.*, 2001). It is possible that many diseases, once considered to be monogenic, will turn out to be complex disorders (Peltonen *et al.*, 2001). It has been suggested that environment and life-style are major contributors to the pathogenesis of complex diseases (Peltonen *et al.*, 2001). In addition, at different stages of pathogenesis of a disease, multiple genes or genetic factors may be involved. For example, the parkin gene is influential in the development of early-onset Parkinson disease, and several genes may influence the development of late-onset Parkinson disease, and so it appears that Parkinson disease is caused by an interaction of genetic and environmental risk factors (Scott et al., 2001).

It is very likely that due to the complexity of the interaction between genetic and environmental risk factors for a disease, even for the same disease, the responsive genes may be different among different affected individuals, whereas the molecular pathways or biological processes affected by the responsive genes might remain the same and persist throughout the individuals with the same disease. The pathway-level or biological process readout may be more consistent than individual genes in these individuals. Therefore, seeking pathway-level consistencies across the affected individuals within the population of the same phenotypic class and pathway-level differences between different phenotypic classes would largely complement approaches relying on the conventional gene-level changes, especially under those circumstances mentioned above. Importantly, by focusing on pathway-level consistencies instead of individual gene-level consistencies, none of the information derived from individual gene-level consistencies is lost, because this information would still be picked up by the analysis method.

6.2.3 Current advances in pathway-level signatures and pathway classification

To move the analysis scheme from the individual gene level to the level of biological processes, several recent methods have used gene modules or gene sets as the basic building blocks for analysis: These methods include some of the gene-set-based methods such as FCS or ORA (Segal et al., 2004, 2005; Huang et al., 2003; Mootha et al., 2003, Lamb et al., 2003). The rationale is that with a modular view of coherent changes in expression in larger modules, it is possible to identify the patterns that are too subtle to be uncovered when considering expression profiles of individual genes in isolation. For example, the GSEA method (Mootha et al., 2003) can detect significant changes even in situations where the expression of individual genes is not significantly different. The underlying patterns with biological themes are only detected when the coherent signal is associated with a high-level entity or module.

Currently, the gene-level paradigm where gene-level differentiated genes or gene-level consistency based on either expression differences or correlations between expression and the phenotype of interest between the two classes, is still conventionally considered as a prerequisite for many analysis schemes, even for group test procedures such as ORA and FCS. Furthermore, FCS methods such as GSEA do not offer a way to assess the enrichment of a pathway or term over a collection of individual samples in a data set. Consequently, GSEA and other FCS methods may miss a particular pathway variation or inconsistency that might characterize a given set of tumour samples (e.g. subtypes of a certain tumour), although some recent methods built on the GSEA algorithm have improved on this limitation with the potential to predict several pathways among individual samples (Tian et al 2005; Edelman et al., 2006).

One module-level analysis scheme obtains a global view of the shared and unique molecular modules underlying human cancer by compiling a 'cancer compendium' from multiple studies and a large collection of biological meaningful gene sets from experimental studies and hand-curated annotations (Segal et al., 2004). The identified gene sets with similar behaviour across arrays were combined into modules, which were used to characterize a variety of clinical conditions (e.g. tumour stages, types, subtypes) with the combination of activated and deactivated modules. In the so-called 'cancer module map', the activation or deactivation of certain modules was shared across multiple tumour types, which was more relevant to the general carcinogenic processes, whereas others were more specific to the tissue types or progression of particular tumours (Segal et al., 2004). This type of analysis claims to be able to increase the ability to identify the signal in microarray data and provide results that are intuitive and more interpretable than simple gene lists. In addition, such a modular approach can be applied to multiple data resources of different biological systems under study to uncover the commonalities and uniqueness of multiple clinical and biological situations. Similar in rationale but different in methodology and algorithm, applying a heatmap type of visualization scheme for embedded biological themes in multiple gene lists (differentially expressed genes, genes with certain profiles or sequence features, etc.) was also similarly implemented in a pathway-level enrichment pattern extraction or analysis pipeline in WPS, as well using enrichment scores that are derived from Fisher's exact test p-values for terms or pathways (Yi et al., 2006, Yi and Stephens, unpublished work on Pathway Pattern Extraction pipeline).

Interestingly, modular approaches have attempted to identify regulatory relationships from genomic data including reconstruction of *cis*-regulatory circuits, detecting targets and discovering new *cis*-elements. Most approaches focusing on regulatory modules assume that member genes are expected to be controlled by similar regulators in a similar fashion (Pilpel et al., 2001; Shen-Orr et al., 2002; Lee et al., 2002). Recent improvements in this method have added evidence from other data sources including factor binding of ChIP-chip array data (Lee et al., 2002) and conservation across species (Lee et al., 2002; Stuart et al., 2003; Pritsker et al., 2004). A model of regulatory modules has been proposed whereby module genes share both similar expression profiles as well as a similar profile of *cis*-elements (Segal et al., 2003a). Thus, a gene's *cis*-element profile determines its module assignment and expression profile. Based on the observation that many regulatory interactions are shared by all members of a gene module, a module-network approach has been proposed to identify modules of co-regulated genes and their shared regulation programme, which specify the expression profile of a module's genes as a function of the expression of the module's regulators (Segal et al., 2003b). This approach has successfully identified functional coherent modules and known regulatory relationships in a yeast expression data set. Noticeably, there is a key limitation for this approach: many regulators are affected post-translationally, and their activity would not be detected in microarray data for gene expression. Interestingly, a newly developed method called SLEPR (Sample-Level Enrichment-based Pathway-Ranking, Yi and Stephens, 2008), which integrates HTP data that measures gene expression, level of post-translational modification, even protein levels, may overcome this limitation. SLEPR is an alternative way to approach the problem of pathway-level consistency in the absence of gene-level consistency. It looks for the underlying biological themes through the pathway-level consistencies based on sample-level enrichment levels of differentiated genes. Similarly, a Pathway Pattern Extraction pipeline, which was implemented in a new version of WPS (Yi et al., 2006), is intended to compare multiple gene lists for their commonality and uniqueness at the pathway level (Yi and Stephens, unpublished work on Pathway Pattern Extraction pipeline). To fulfil this goal, this analysis pipeline used list-level enrichment levels of pathways/terms that are derived from Fisher's exact test p-values for different gene lists to look for the patterned pathways such as common or unique pathways/terms that are enriched either consistently among the lists or specifically in one list but not in others (Yi and Stephens, unpublished work on Pathway Pattern Extraction pipeline).

By taking a different direction to generate experimental data under the conditions of knowing whether a known pathway is active or not prior to data analysis, a distinct method pursues gene expression signatures that are experimentally generated to specifically reflect the status of the pathway as either active or inactive for various oncogenic signalling pathways. One example was to use quiescent cells, in which many of the pathways of interest (e.g. apoptosis pathways, proliferation-related pathways) will be inactive (Huang et al., 2003). Thus, individual pathways are then activated in these cells by means of expressing a relevant gene through infection with an adenovirus (Huang et al., 2003). This experimental approach can isolate the effects of single pathway activation and then generate corresponding expression signatures or pathway signatures that reflect this process. Practically, these profiles are represented as metagenes, which mathematically consist of collections of gene expression values in aggregate form, characteristic of an experimentally defined condition including pathway activation in this case (Bild et al., 2006a). Alternative approaches to this same method include the use of mouse tumour models (Sweet-Cordero et al., 2005) or cells stably transformed by the expression of an oncogene or the loss of a tumour suppressor gene (Singh et al., 2001). These signatures provide a way to assess the status of the pathway by evaluating the extent to which the signatures identified from the training set is represented in an individual sample. The probabilities of pathway activation are estimated with internal validation that defines the pathway signature using an external set of samples, which are further visualized in a heatmap with colour cues to indicate whether the probability is high or low (Bild et al., 2006a). A high probability would indicate the corresponding sample may be more likely to express such a pathway signature. Such experimentally defined pathway signatures provide an opportunity to identify patterns of pathway de-regulation within individual samples, e.g. identify subclasses of tumours with common properties (Bild et al., 2006a). It has been shown that identifying patterns of pathway deregulation helps to better categorize cancer patients in that certain subgroups of patients, who are identified by unique pathway patterns, are more likely to suffer a recurrence of disease than others (Bild et al., 2006a, 2006b). Furthermore, there is a clear relationship between the prediction of pathway deregulation and sensitivity to the respective therapeutic target, which promises to link pathway predictions with drug sensitivity (Bild et al., 2006b).

A confounding discovery from these studies is the observation that just as genes do not act in a vacuum, pathways are similarly interconnected, with intracellular feedback loops as well as autocrine and paracrine signalling mechanisms complicating the interpretation of these data. Analysis of complex diseases such as cancer have revealed initiating pathway perturbations followed by the accumulation of additional mutations in additional pathways that further disarm the individual's ability to respond to and control tumour growth and spread through the system. It is likely that as these multiple pathways become better understood, their interactions will become apparent.

Another method similar in principle but different in methodology extends pathway signature methods one step further by combining gene signatures derived from expression data with regulatory motif analysis using an enrichment-based method. The method attempts to discover activated or inactivated signalling pathways (Liu and Ringer, 2007). This approach is able to identify pathways deregulated in gene expression signatures by viewing these signatures as a collection of target genes of the transcription factors that mediate the pathways, and appears to be better than the EASE (Hosack et al., 2003) and GSEA (Mootha et al., 2003) methods in identifying expected pathways in data sets with known pathway activation (Liu and Ringer, 2007).

More recently, a new method (Efroni et al., 2007), which is based on network structure information or interdependence of a network and the observation of co-expression of a set of genes is able to choose a miniset of pathways that can classify phenotypes. The method also considers the probability of being in a 'down' or 'up' state for genes within a data set and calculates the pathway consistency scores for each interaction in a pathway and for pathway activity scores. This method, termed the Efroni method, has some similarities to the modular method (Segal et al., 2004) mentioned above. However, there are some obvious distinctions. First of all, the modular method uses biological modules that were internally defined within the paper, whereas the Efroni method uses externally defined canonical pathways independent of the data that they were used with. Secondly, the Efroni method is probably the only pathway-level classification method so far that makes explicit use of the network structure including interconnections of the nodes that exist between genes that form the biological modules, although substructure information from the network has been used initially in a qualitative approach of metabolic pathway analysis using elementary modes, which allows the study of the possible behaviour of a system from only the structure of the network (Peres et al., 2006). The calculated pathway scores of activity and consistency are based on network structure and their directive relations (e.g. inhibition and promotion), which are features or substructure information of network information (Efroni et al., 2007). The Enrichment score-based Pathway Pattern Extraction method in the newly developed pathway analysis pipeline (Yi and Stephens, unpublished work on Pathway Pattern Extraction pipeline) and the SLEPR method (Yi and Stephens, 2008) also attempts to use a pathway-level metric similar to that used by the Efroni method (although a different metric is derived from pathway enrichment scores instead of pathway consistency or activity scores derived from network information) to represent an individual sample or gene list that allows for pathway-level pattern extraction or pathway ranking.

Another method called LeFE developed very recently, which implemented a machine learning algorithm based on Random Forest Sampling, was able to capture complex, system-oriented information for prediction of functional signatures (Eichler et al., 2007). LeFE determines for each category or gene set whether its genes are more important as predictors (variables) than a set of randomly sampled negative controlled genes. Although the LeFE method could not claim to be 'better' than the GSEA method, it does directly handle problem types (multiple class, continuous-valued signature, small gene sets) not handled by many other related gene-set based methods (Eichler et al., 2007).

In order to show the differences between conventional gene-level methods and pathway-level analysis methods, we specifically used our newly developed SLEPR method and Pathway Pattern Extraction pipeline implemented in the new version of the WPS program (Yi et al., 2006; Yi and Stephens, unpublished work on SLEPR method and Pathway Pattern Extraction pipeline) as an example for a more detailed graphical illustration in Fig. 6.1. As shown in Fig. 6.1(a), the conventional gene-level methods primarily consider sample-level changes with gene-level consistency, which is vulnerable to biological variation in the population and even experimental variation in the data. In contrast, SLEPR (Yi and Stephens, 2008) relies on the feasible assumption that pathway-level consistencies across individual samples and individuals in population might be more persistent or penetrant than consistencies of individual genes, which appeared to be highly likely in terms of its validity (Fig. 6.1(b)). Pathway Pattern Extraction pipeline (Yi and Stephens, 2008) is intended to extract the pathway-level patterns beyond individual gene in the gene lists under study, which may obtain patterns that could be missing from the gene-level methods (Fig. 6.1(b)).

There exists a major difference between the conventional gene-level based group test methods and the SLEPR method. Conventional gene-level based methods directly use cross-sample evaluation for differentiated genes or ranking the genes such as GSEA method. In contrast, SLEPR uses cross-sample evaluation to get sample-wise potentially 'changed' genes of individual samples, or sample-level differentiated genes, followed by cross-sample evaluation of pathway-level enrichment levels for differentiated pathways. Such operational differences reflected the differences in concepts and rationales of these methods, which would lead to quite different outcomes in analysis of data derived from many of the complicated studies. Using three previously analysed publicly available sample data sets and side-by-side comparison with the GSEA method, the SLEPR method was able to not only reproduce the previous insights with more robust statistics, but significantly extend the observations made by the GSEA method with additional insights (Yi and Stephens, 2008). The SLEPR method was designed to provide an alternative way to compensate for, or even overcome, the limitation that may be encountered by group test methods such as FCS, which rely on or start with a gene-level paradigm. Furthermore, since sample-level differentiated genes should capture individual variation or specificity and also maintain class-wise differences of each individual sample, data sets measuring changes at different levels of regulation of genes, including transcription, protein expression, and phosphorylation occurring in the same individual samples, all HTP data measuring these changes in the systems biology era can be integrated and included in SLEPR method.

6.3   Potentials of pathway-based analysis for integrative discovery

Over the years, pathway-based analysis has drawn more and more attention from the research community. This is probably, at first glance, due to its great analytical abilities and intuitive ways of interpreting high-throughput data in a biological context, which appears to be the most attractive to biological researchers themselves due to its ease in interpretation and comprehensiveness. But in the prospective view of the bioinformatics field, more importantly, this is also driven by the expectation that biological network/pathways could provide a mathematical matrix enriched with biological relevances such as detailed gene–gene interaction relationships for statistical analysis at a more comprehensive level. Such settings are getting closer in nature to the reality of biological systems with extreme complexities and would largely facilitate the processes of integrative discovery.

As illustrated in Fig. 6.2, on top of pathways that consist of functionally connected genes, a biological network can be viewed as logically linked pathways with conjunctions of critical genes or hubs, which may play multiple roles within multiple pathways or biological processes with different biological outputs and functions. Such a gene-pathway-network architecture becomes increasingly promising for providing an excellent environment and context for seeking biological themes. As described earlier, many currently available tools have used such contexts to directly and simply map the derived differentiated genes or gene signatures from the data into such network/pathways in a variety of ways for the purpose of data visualization and seeking biological relevancies and significance from the neighbourhood of those chosen genes. Such an intuitive method is the most popular approach to the conventional pathway-based analysis scheme. However, the demands for integrative-types of analysis for discovery have dramatically increased over recent years as a variety of data types as well as massive amounts of data derived from numerous improved or novel technologies in era of systems biology, including microarray data (conventional expression

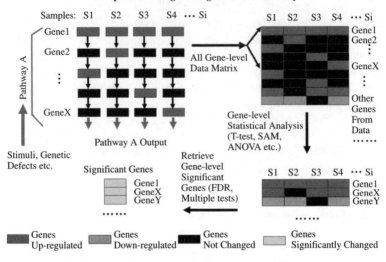

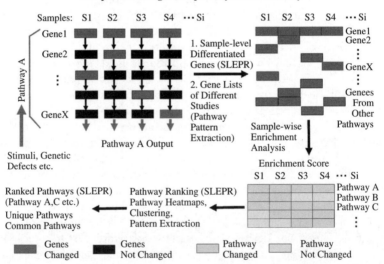

FIG. 6.1: Comparison of conventional gene-level methods and SLEPR or Pathway-level Pattern Extraction. Graphical display and comparison of the brief procedures for analysis using conventional gene-level methods vs. SLEPR or Pathway-level Pattern Extraction methods. Pathway A was shown as an example pathway among the whole biological system, in which many of its involved genes were changed triggered by biological stimuli, or genetic defects in disease states. The conventional gene-level methods and SLEPR or Pathway-level Pattern Extraction pipeline processed the genes from pathway A

array, exon array, CGH array, miRNA array, SNP array), proteomic data (antibody/protein array, mass spectrometry), protein-protein interaction data (e.g. high-throughput two-hybrid data), protein-DNA interaction data (e.g. ChIP-chip for transcription factor-promoter interaction, genome-wide methylation etc.), genome-wide post-translational modification data (e.g. electron transfer dissociation or ETD), and many other in-silicon data such as transcription binding site prediction, miRNA target prediction, data or text mining from literature have emerged. In addition, as the setting of network/pathways with enriched biological contexts opens up a new view and field as the possible new matrix and inputs for statistical and bioinformatics analysis methods and algorithms, the new needs for method integration in the realm of networks and pathways will continue to rise, which will lead to the next generation of analysis schemes. As a consequence, data and method integration within the context of biological networks/pathways will become a major challenge for pathway-based analysis in the era of systems biology.

Figure 6.1 *Continued*

---

as well as other pathways in different ways even for the same biological situations under study. (a) Within a typical procedure of gene-level methods, all measured data of each sample in study are usually put together into a gene-level data matrix, and then a statistical analysis method (T-test, SAM, ANOVA, etc.) is applied to all genes of the matrix to retrieve the gene-level significant genes based on one or more statistical parameters (e.g. p-value, fold change, FDR, etc.). Significant genes usually behave with a greater gene-level consistency across samples in each population of contrasted classes. (b) For the SLEPR procedure, all measured data of each sample are used to derive the sample-level differentiated genes, which represent genes for each sample that are expressed differentiatelly compared to the rest of samples in the population (see SLEPR manuscript for details, each sample will get a corresponding list of sample-level differentiated genes). Then, sample-level differentiated genes (for SLEPR) or all gene lists of different studies (for Pathway-level Pattern Extraction pipeline) were used to perform sample-wise enrichment analysis against each of functional annotation categories (e.g. GO terms, GSEA annotation terms, or Biocarta Pathways, etc.). The derived enrichment scores (ES) of each term in the chosen functional category for each gene list were combined into an enrichment score matrix. Then pathway ranking (for SLEPR), pathway ES heatmaps, clustering, and pattern extraction (for Pathway-level Pattern Extraction) will be applied to this ES matrix to get significantly ranked pathways (SLEPR), unique pathways, common pathways (for Pathway-level Pattern Extraction), respectively. Genes that are associated with these pathways or terms can be retrieved further within the Pathway Pattern Extraction pipeline. See Plate 4.

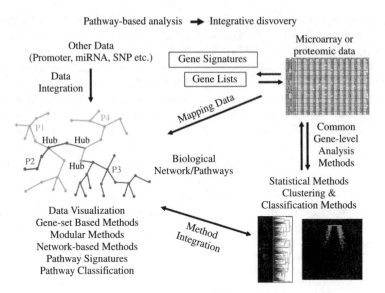

FIG. 6.2: Prospects of pathway-based analysis: integrative discovery. In the era of systems biology with accumulation of massive data and numerous statistical and bioinformatics methods available, pathway-based analysis may become a pioneer for integrative discovery. It will evolve from a simple analysis scheme of mapping gene lists into a biological network for data visualization to look for biological relevance and significance from the neighbourhood of those chosen genes, into the integrative discovery scheme through integration of both data and method sides using the biological network/pathways as a common ground. Such evolution includes: from gene-based methods (e.g. gene signature), to pathway-level based method (e.g. gene set, modular methods, network-based method; pathway signatures and pathway classification), to more integrative methods. The nodes in the network are genes and the lines indicate either physical or genetic connections among the genes. P1–P4 are examples of pathways existing inside the network, with different colours denoting different pathways. The nodes labelled as 'Hub' are genes involved in multiple pathways, which may play multiple functional roles.

There are many obvious advantages making this transition. First, with the help of functional connections of genes and pathways in biological networks, which could be interfered or impaired from diseases and other conditions, we could allow the integration of different data that look into the system at different levels and angles of the involved genes with a more or close-to complete scale or genome-wide scale. Such integration would provide multiple-dimensional views of the biological system under study that may be especially and in fact desperately needed for dissecting the most complicated systems or biological systems we deal with. Although it may be overwhelming at first, this additional information, once incorporated and integrated into the analysis, could represent a missing link to generating scientific hypotheses about the cause, treatment or progression of a complex disease or condition.

Secondly, with knowing genes or groups of genes working together as a unit in a pathway or a gene set scope and in a larger scale within a network for their interdependences and interactions with other genes and pathways through network hub genes, a possible weighted matrix of these genes that accounts for their contributions to the system as a network can be captured and used as additional inputs for integration of analysis methods and algorithms for a new analysis scheme that has yet to be explored. Preliminary efforts (Efroni et al., 2007; Lu et al., 2007; Ulitsky and Shamir, 2007) in such a direction have been made recently as discussed earlier.

Thirdly, the organization of our studied system into a gene-pathway-network hierarchical structure made it possible to move from our analysis scheme from gene-level, to pathway or gene-set-level, and even to subnetwork or network level for different biological systems with different levels of complexity. For example, some rare diseases could be caused by a single gene in some populations with less variation. The gene-level approach can be powerful and has proven to be successful in such circumstances. However, as we mentioned earlier, some complex diseases such as cancers already were known having multiple genes involved and were different in subtypes and populations with different genetic background. The underlying pathogenesis mechanisms of such complex diseases may not be easily dissected and uncovered by conventional gene-level methods. Instead, pathway-level methods may have a better chance when they face up to the complexities of such diseases. Initial efforts have been made to use pathway or gene set signatures and classification to characterize different stages, types, and/or subtypes of diseases especially on cancer, which has been discussed earlier (Segal et al., 2004; Efroni et al., 2007; Yi and Stephens, unpublished work). The integration from both sides of data and methods on top of the biological network/pathways would largely improve such efforts with the further help from information regarding the structure of a network and the interconnection of nodes or genes within a network. To bring together relevant data from all sources, and all the available statistical or bioinformatics analysis methodologies and algorithms under one roof of gene-pathway-network environment, pathway-based analysis approach would yield a better chance to really evolve into the most powerful analysis scheme for integrative discovery.

6.4 Conclusions

Over the course of their relatively short history, microarray analysis tools have evolved into two principal classes – tools for normalizing and clustering data and tools for placing the data into the context of their associated biology. More recently, the latter set of tools has been undergoing a dramatic enhancement in capabilities through conceptual expansion of both the methodologies they employ, but also the expansion of the sources of biological data that they utilize to gain biological insights. As the volume of data produced in any HTP experiments is large and complex, visualization and analysis of these results has also evolved from early generation of lists of differentially expressed genes to visualization of complex networks of interacting entities or terms to much more comprehensive ways for integrated discovery. The opportunity now exists to identify and prioritize target pathways and other biologically significant information from relatively routine analysis methods. In addition, classifier and biomarker identification for particular phenotypes has also become an important and increasingly reachable capability. As more and more information about the complexity and diversity of biological systems is understood, these tools for analysis of complex data will continue to improve and aid in the goal of disease detection and treatment.

The common gene-level statistical approaches and gene-based classification methods have encountered some limitations especially as a better understanding of the complexity of biological systems and diseases in the post-genomic era has emerged. The pathway signatures and pathway classifiers may provide an alternative way to compensate for, or even overcome the limitations that may be encountered by analysis methods based on the gene-level paradigm. The pathway-level paradigm represents a new way to analyse high throughput data through pathway signatures, pathway-level patterns, pathway-level consistencies, which have been proven to be increasingly effective in uncovering biological themes. In addition, pathway signatures and pathway classifiers derived from data sets for a particular study may turn out to be more generic than gene signatures and classifiers and may be more useful when applied to diagnosing complicated diseases and dissecting biological systems. Also, conceptualizing signalling and regulatory 'modules' rather than individual genes may yield insights into comparative species differences in the different pharmacological responses seen by different species to a particular therapeutic treatment regimen. In addition, biological changes at different levels of regulation, including transcription, protein expression, and phosphorylation occurring in the same individual samples, which can now be measured with all types of HTP technologies as they become increasly feasible, could be more likely integrated for discovery of underlying biological themes under the context of pathways, gene set, biological modules, as well as complicated networks.

References

Al-Shahrour, F., Díaz-Uriarte, R., and Dopazo, J. (2004). FatiGO: a web tool for finding significant associations of Gene Ontology terms with groups of genes. *Bioinformatics*, **20**, 578–80.

Baitaluk, M., Qian, X., Godbole, S., Raval, A., Ray, A., and Gupta, A. (2006). PathSys: integrating molecular interaction graphs for systems biology. *BMC Bioinformatics*, **7**, 55.

Bild, A. H., Guang Yao, Jeffrey T. Chang, Quanli Wang, Anil Potti, Dawn Chasse, Mary-Beth Joshi, David Harpole, Johnathan M. Lancaster, Andrew Berchuck, John A. Olson, Jr, Jeffrey R. Marks, and Holly K. Dressman

(2006a). Mike West and Joseph R. Nevins. Oncogenic pathway signatures in human cancers as a guide to targeted therapies. *Nature*, **439**, 353–357.

Bild, A. H., Anil Potti, and Joseph R. Nevins (2006b). Opinion: Linking oncogenic pathways with therapeutic opportunities. *Nature Reviews Cancer*, **6**, 735–741.

Boorsma, A., Foat, B. C., Vis, D., Klis, F., and Bussemaker, H. J. (2005). T-profiler: scoring the activity of predefined groups of genes using gene expression data. *Nucleic Acids Res*, **33**, web server issue W592–W595.

Breiman, L. Random forest. *Machine Learning* 2001, **45**, 5–32.

Breitkreutz, B. J., Stark, C., and Tyers, M. (2003). Osprey: a network visualization system. *Genome Biology*, **4(3)**, R22.

Cartharius, K., Frech, K., Grote, K., Klocke, B., Haltmeier, M., Klingenhoff, A., Frisch, M., Bayerlein, M., and Werner, T. (2005) MatInspector and beyond: promoter analysis based on transcription factor binding sites. *Bioinformatics*, **21(13)**, 2933–42.

Cary, M., Bader, G., and Sander, C. (2005). Pathway information for systems biology. *FEBS Letters*, **579(8)**, 1815–1820.

Chen, J. J., Tsai, C.-A., Tzeng, S. L., and Chen, C.-H. (2007). Gene slection with multiple ordering crieterria. *BMC Bioinformatics*, **8**, 74.

Cho, J. H., Lee, D., Park, J. H., and Lee, I. B. (2004). Gene slection and classification from miroarray data using kernel machine. *FEBS Letters*, **571**, 93–98.

Chu T.-M., Weir, B., and Wolfinger, R. (2002). A systematic statistical linear modeling approach to oligonucleotide array experiments. *Mathematical Bioscience*, **176**, 35–51.

Curtisa, K. R., Oresicb, M., and Vidal-Puiga, A. (2005). Pathways to the analysis of microarray data. *Trends in Biotechnology*, **23(8)**, 429–435.

Dahlquist, K. D., Salomonis, N., Vranizan, K., Lawlor, S. C., and Conklin, B. R. (2002). GenMAPP, a new tool for viewing and analyzing microarray data on biological pathways, *Nat. Genetics*, **31(1)**, 19–20.

Damian, D. and Gorfine, M. (2004). Statistical concerns about the GSEA procedure. *Nat. Genetics*, **36(7)**, 663.

Dennis, G. Jr, Sherman, B. T., Hosack, D. A., Yang, J., Gao, W., Lane, H. C., and Lempicki, R. A. (2003). DAVID: Database for Annotation, Visualization, and Integrated Discovery. *Genome Biology*, **4(5)**, P3.

Dobbin, K. K. and Simon, R. M. (2007). Sample size planning for developing classifiers using high-dimensional DNA microarray data. *Biostatistics*, **8**, 101–117.

Dohr, S., Klingenhoff, A., Maier, H., Hrabé de Angelis, M., Werner, T., and Schneider, R. (2005). Linking disease-associated genes to regulatory networks via promoter organization. *Nucleic Acids Research*, **33**, 864–872.

Draghici, S., Kuklin, A., Hoff, B., and Shams, S. (2001). Experimental design, analysis of variance and slide quality assessment in gene expression arrays. *Current Opinions in Drug Discovery and Development*, **4**, 332–7.

Draghici, S., Khatri, P., Martins, R. P., Ostermeier, G. C., and Krawetz, S. A. (2003a). Global functional profiling of gene expression. *Genomics*, **81(2)**, 98–104.

Draghici, S., Kulaeva, O., Hoff, B., Petrov, A., Shams, S., and Tainsky, M. A. (2003b). Noise sampling method: an ANOVA approach allowing robust selection of differentially regulated genes measured by DNA microarrays. *Bioinformatics*, **19**, 1348–59.

Dudoit, S., Fridlyand, J., and Speed, T. P. (2002). Comparison of discrimination methods for the classification of tumors using gene expression data. *Journal of the American Statistical Association*, **97**, 77–87.

Edelman, E., Porrello, A., Guinney, J., Balakumaran, B., Bild, A., Febbo, P. G., and Mukherjee, S. (2006). Analysis of sample set enrichment scores: assaying the enrichment of sets of genes for individual samples in genome-wide expression profiles. *Bioinformatics*, **22(14)**, e108–16.

Efroni, S., Schaefer, C. F., and Beutow, K. H. (2007). Identification of key processes underlying cancer phenotypes using biological pathway analysis. *Plos ONE*, **2(5)**, e425.

Eichler, G. S., Reimers, M., Kane, D., and Weinstein, J. N. (2007). The LeFE algorithm: embracing the complexity of gene expression in the interpretation of microarray data. *Genome Biology*, **8**, R187.

Eisen, M. B., Spellman, P. T., Brown, P. O., and Botstein, D. (1998). Clustering analysis and display of genome-wide expression patterns. *Proceedings of the National Academy of Science, USA*, **95**, 14863–14868.

Goeman, J. J., van de Geer, S. A., de Kort, F., van Houwelingen, H. C. (2004). A global test for groups of genes: testing association with a clincal outcome. *Bioinformatics*, **20**, 93–99.

Golub, T. R., Slonim, D. K., Tamayo, P., Huard, C., Gaasenbeek, M., Mesirov, J. P., Coller, H., Loh, M. L., Downing, J. R., Caligiuri, M. A., Bloomfield, C. D., and Lander, E. S. (1999). Molecular classification of cancer: Class discovery and class prediction by gene expression monitoring. *Science*, **286(5439)**, 531–537.

Grosu, P., Townsend, J. P., Hartl, D. L., and Cavalieri, D. (2002). Pathway Processor: A tool for integrating whole-genome expression results into metabolic networks. *Genome Research*, **12(7)**, 1121–1126.

Guyon, I., Weston, J., Barnhill, S., and Vapnik, V. (2002). Gene selection for cancer classification using support vector machines. *Machine Learning*, **46**, 389–422.

Hartigan, J. A. and Wong, M. A. (1979). A k-means clustering algorithm. *Applied Statistics*, **28**, 100–108.

Hosack D. A., Dennis, Jr G., Sherman, B. T., Lane, H. C., and Lempicki, R. A. (2003). Identifying biological themes within lists of genes with EASE. *Genome Biology*, **4**, R70.

Hsieh, W.-P., Chu, T.-M., Wolfinger, R. D., and Gibson, G. (2003). Mixed-model reanalysis of primate data suggested tissue and species biases in oligonucleotide-based gene expression profiles. *Genetics*, **165**, 747–757.

Hu, Z., Mellor, J., Wu, J., and DeLisi, C. (2004). VisANT: an online visualization and analysis tool for biological interaction data. *BMC Bioinformatics*, **5**, 17.

Huang, E., Ishida, S., Pittman, J., Dressman, H., Bild, A., Kloos, M., D'Amico, M., Pestell, R. G., West, M., and Nevins, J. R. (2003). Gene expression phenotypic models that predict the activity of oncogenic pathways. *Nature Genetics*, **34**, 226–230.

Hucka, M., Finney, A., Sauro, H. M., Bolouri, H., Doyle, J. C., Kitano, H., Arkin, A. P., Bornstein, B. J., Bray, D., Cornish-Bowden, A., Cuellar, A. A., Dronov, S., Gilles, E. D., Ginkel, M., Gor, V., Goryanin, I. I., Hedley, W. J., Hodgman, T. C., Hofmeyr, J. H., Hunter, P. J., Juty, N. S., Kasberger, J. L., Kremling, A., Kummer, U., Le Novere, N., Loew, L. M., Lucio, D., Mendes, P., Minch, E., Mjolsness, E. D., Nakayama, Y., Nelson, M. R., Nielsen, P. F., Sakurada, T., Schaff, J. C., Shapiro, B. E., Shimizu, T. S., Spence, H. D., Stelling, J., Takahashi, K., Tomita, M., Wagner, J., and Wang, J., SBML Forum, (2003). The systems biology markup language (SBML): a medium for representation and exchange of biochemical network models. *Bioinformatics*, **19(4)**, 524–31.

Jain, N., Ley, K., Thatte, J., O'Connell, M., and Lee, J. K. (2003). Local pooled error test for identifying differentially expressed genes with a small number of replicated microarrays. *Bioinformatics*, **19(15)**, 1945–51.

Kanehisa, M., Goto, S., Kawashima, S., and Nakaya, A. (2002). The KEGG databases at GenomeNet. *Nucleic Acids Research*, **30**, 42–46

Karp, P. D., Paley, S., and Romero, P. (2002). The Pathway Tools Software, *Bioinformatics*, **18**, S225–32.

Kerr, M. K., Martin, M., and Churchill, G. (2000). Analysis of variance for gene expression microarray data. *Journal of Computational Biology*, **7**, 819–837.

Kim, S.-Y. and Volsky, D. (2005) PAGE: Parametric Analysis of Gene Set Enrichment. *BMC Bioinformatics*, **6**, 144.

Lamb, L., Ramaswamy, S., Ford, H. L., Contreras, B., Martinez, R. V., Kittrell, F. S., Zahnow, C. A., Patterson, N., Golub, T. R., and Ewen, M. E. (2003). A mechanism of cyclin D1 action encoded in the patterns of gene expression in human cancer. *Cell*, **114**, 323–334.

Lee, T. I., Rinaldi, N. J., Robert, F., Odom, D. T., Bar-Joseph, Z., Gerber, G. K., Hannett, N. M., Harbison, C. T., Thompson, C. M., Simon, I., Zeitlinger, J., Jennings, E. G., Murray, H. L., Gordon, B. D., Ren, B., Wyrick, J. J., Tagne, J. B., Volkert, T. L., Fraenkel, E., Gifford, D. K., and Young, R. A. (2002). Transcriptional Regulatory Networks in Saccharomyces cerevisiae. *Science*, **298**, 799–804.

Li, L., Weinberg, C., Darden, T., and Padersen, L. (2001). Gene selection for sample classification based on gene expression data: study of sensitivity to choice of parameters of the GA/KNN method. *Bioinformatics*, **17**, 1131–1142.

Liu, Y. and Ringner, M. (2007). Revealing signaling pathway deregulation by using gene expression signatures and regulatory motif analysis. *Genome Biology*, **8(5)**, R77.

Lloyd, C. M., Halstead, M. D., and Nielsen, P. F. (2004). CellML: its future, present and past. *Progress in Biophysics and Molecular Biology*, **85**, 433–450.

Lu, X., Jain, V. V., Finn, P. W., and Perkins, D. L. (2007). Hubs in biological interaction networks exhibit low changes in expression in experimental asthma. *Molecular Systems Biology*, **3**, 98.

Luyf, A. C. M., de Cast, J., and van Kampen, A. H. C. (2002). Visualizing metabolic activity on a genome-wide scale. *Bioinformatics*, **18**, 813–818.

MAQC Consortium (2006). The MicroArray Quality Control (MAQC) project shows inter- and intraplatform reproducibility of gene expression measurements. *Nature Biotechnology*, **24**, 1151–1169

Manoli, T., Gretz, N., Grone, H.-J., Kenzelmann, M., Elis, R., and Brors, B. (2006). Group testing for pathway analysis improves comparability of different microarray datasets. *Bioinformatics*, **22**, 2500–2506.

Michiels, S., Koscielny, S., and Hill, C. (2005). Prediction of cancer outcome with microarrays: a multiple random validation strategy. *The Lancet*, **365**, 488–492.

Moon, H., Ahn, H., Kodell, R. L., Lin, C. J., Beak, S., and Chen, J. J. (2006). Classification methods for the development of genomic signatures from high-dimensional data. *Genome Biology*, **7**, R121.

Mootha, V. K., Lindgren, C. M., Eriksson, K. F., Subramanian, A., Sihag, S., Lehar, J., Puigserver, P., Carlsson, E., Ridderstrale, M., Laurila, E. et al. (2003). PGC-1-responsive genes involved in oxidative phosphorylation are coordinately downregulated in human diabetes. *Nature Genetics*, **34**, 267–273.

Nadon, R. and Shoemaker, J. (2002). Statistical issues with microarrays: pro-cessing and analysis. *Trends in Genetics*, **18**, 265–71.

Nakao, M., Bono, H., Kawashima, S., Kamiya, T., Sato, K., Goto, S., and Kanehisa, M. (1999). Genome-scale gene expression analysis and pathway reconstruction in KEGG. *Genome Information Series Workshop*, **10**, 94–103.

Nikitin, A., Egorov, S., Daraselia, N., and Mazo, I. (2003). Pathway studio – the analysis and navigation of molecular networks. *Bioinformatics*, **19(16)**, 2155–7.

Ntzani, E. E. and Loannidis, J. P. (2003). Predictive ability of DNA microarrays for cancer outcomes and correlates: an empirical assessment. *The Lancet*, **362**, 1439–44.

Pavlidis, P., Qin, J., Arango, V., Mann, J. J., and Sibille, E. (2004). Using the gene ontology for microarray data mining: a comparison of methods and application to age effects in human prefrontal cortex. *Neurochemical Research*, **29**, 1213–1222.

Pavlidis, P. (2003). Using ANOVA for gene selection from microarray studies of nervous system. *Methods*, **31**, 282–89.

Pavlidis, P., Lewis, D. P., and Noble, W. S. (2002). Exploring gene expression data with class scores. *Pacific Symposium on Biocomputing*, **7**, 474–485.

Peltonen, L. and McKusick, V. A. (2001). Genomics and medicine: dissecting human disease in postgenomic era. *Science*, **291**, 1224–1229.

Peres, S., Beurton-Aimar, M., and Mazat, J. P. (2006). Pathway classification of TCA cycle. *IEE Proceedings Systems Biology*, **153(5)**, 369–371.

Perket, J. M. (2006). Six things you won't find in the MAQC. *The Scientist*, **20**, 68–72.

Pilpel, Y., Priya Sudarsanam, P., George, M., and Church, G. M. (2001). Identifying regulatory networks by combinatorial analysis of promoter elements. *Nature Genetics*, **29**, 153–159.

Pritsker, M., Liu, Y. C., Beer, M. A., and Tavazoie. (2004). Whole-genome discovery of transcription factor binding sites by network-level conservation. *Genome Research*, **14(1)**, 99–108.

Reiter, L. T., Potocki, L., Chien, S., Gribskov, M., and Bier, E. (2001). A systematic analysis of human disease-associated genes sequences in *Drosophila* melanogaster. *Genome Research*, **11**, 1114–1125.

Rhodes, D. R. and Chinnaiyan, A. M. (2005). Integrative analysis of the cancer transcriptiome. *Nature Genetics*, Suppl. **37**, S31–37.

Scherf, M., Epple, A., and Werner, T. (2005). The next generation of literature analysis: integration of genomic analysis into text mining. *Briefings in Bioinformatics*, **6(3)**, 287–97.

Scott, W. K., Nance, M. A., Watts, R. L., Hubble, J. P., Koller, W. C., Lyons, K., Pahwa, R., Stern, M., Colcher, A., Hiner, B. C. *et al.* (2001). Complete genomic screen in Parkinson's disease: evidence for multiple genes. *JAMA*, **286**(18), 2239–2244.

Segal, E., Barash, Y., Simon, I., Friedman, N., and Koller, D. (2003a). Genome-wide discovery of transcriptional modules from DNA sequence and gene expression. *Bioinformatics*, 19 Suppl. **1**, i273–i282.

Segal, E., Michael Shapira, M., Regev, A., Pe'er, D., Botstein, D., Koller, D., and Friedman, N. (2003b). Module networks: identifying regulatory modules and their condition-specific regulators from gene expression data. *Nature Genetics*, **34**, 166–176.

Segal, E., Friedman, N., Koller, D., and Regev, A. (2004). A module map showing conditional activity of expression modules in cancer. *Nature Genetics*, **36**, 1090–1098.

Segal, E., Friedman, N., Kaminski, N., Regev, A., and Koller, D. (2005). From signatures to models: understanding cancer using microarrays. *Nature Genetics*, **37**, S38–S45.

Shannon, P., Markiel, A., Ozier, O., Baliga, N. S., Wang, J. T., Ramage, D., Amin, N., Schwikowski, B., and Ideker, T. (2003). Cytoscape: A software environment for integrated models of biomolecular interaction networks. *Genome Research*, **13**, 2498–2504.

Shen-Orr, S. S., Milo, R., Mangan, S., and Alon, U. (2002). Network motifs in the transcriptional regulation network of Escherichia coli. *Nature Genetics*, **31**, 64–68.

Singh, D., Febbo, P. G., Ross, K., Jackson, D. G., Manola, J., Ladd, C., Tamayo, P., Renshaw, A. A., D'Amico, A. V., Richie, J. P., Lander, E. S., Loda, M., Kantoff, P. W., Golub, T. R., and Sellers, W. R. (2001). Gene expression correlates of clinical prostate cancer behavior. *Cancer Cell*, **1**, 203–209.

Smyth, G. K., Yang, Y. H., and Speed, T. P. (2003). Statistical issues in microarray data analysis. *Methods in Molecular Biology*, **224**, 111–136.

Smyth, G. K. (2005). Limma: linear models for microarray data. In *Bioinformatics and Computational Biology Solutions using R and Bioconductor*, Springer, New York, pp. 397–420.

Storey, J. D., and Tibshirani, R. (2003). Statistical significance for genomewide studies. *Proceedings of the National Academy of Science, USA*, **100**, 9440–9445.

Stuart, J. M., Segal, E., Koller, D., and Kim, S. K. (2003). A Gene-coexpression network for global discovery of conserved genetic modules. *Science*, **302**, 249–255.

Subramanian, A., Tamayo, P., Mootha, V., Mukherjee, S., Ebert, B. L., Gillette, M. A., Paulovich, A., Pomeroy, S., Golub, T. R., Lander, E., and Mesirov, J. P. (2005). Gene set enrichment analysis: a knowledge-based approach for interpreting genome-wide expression profiles. *Proceedings of the National Academy of Science, USA*, **102**, 15545–15550.

Suderman, M. and Hallett, M. (2007). Tools for visually exploring biological networks. *Bioinformatics*, **23**, 2651–9 [Epub ahead of print].

Sweet-Cordero, A., Mukherjee, S., Subramanian, A., You, H., Roix, J. J., Ladd-Acosta, C., Mesirov, J., Golub, T. R., and Jacks, T. (2005). An oncogenic KRAS2 expression signature identified by cross-species gene-expression analysis. *Nature Genetics*, **37**, 48–55.

Tamayo, P., Slonim, D., Mesirov, J., Zhu, Q., Kitareewan, S., Dmitrovsky, E., Lander, E. S., and Golub, T. R. (1999). Interpreting patterns of gene expression with self-organizing maps: Methods and application to hematopoietic differentiation. *Proceedings of the National Academy of Science, USA*, **96**, 2907–2912.

Tao, H., Bausch, C., Richmond, C., Blattner, F. R., and Conway, T. (1999). Functional genomics: expression analysis of Escherichia coli growing on minimal and rich media. *Journal of Bacteriology*, **181**, 6425–40.

Tian, L., Greenberg, S. A., Kong, S. W., Altschuler, J., Kohane, I. S., and Park, P. J. (2005). Discovering statistically significant pathways in expression profiling studies. *Proceedings of the National Academy of Science, USA*, **102**, 13544–13549.

Tibshirani (1996). Bias, variance and prediction error for classification rules, University of Toronto, Department of Statistics Technical Report, November 1996 (also available at www-stat.standofrd.edu/~tibs).

Tibshirani, R., Hastie, T., Narasimhan, B., and Chu, G. (2002). Diagnosis of multiple cancer types by shrunken centroids of gene expression. *Proceedings of the National Academy of Science, USA*, **99(10)**, 6567–6572.

Tomfohr, J., Lu, J., and Kepler, T. B. (2005). Pathway level analysis of gene expression using singular value decomposition. *BMC Bioinformatics*, **6**, 225.

Tusher, V. G., Tibshirani, R., and Chu, G. (2001). Significance analysis of microarrays applied to ionizing radiation response. *Proceedings of the National Academy of Science, USA*, **98**, 5116–5121.

Ulitsky, I. and Shamir, R. (2007). Identification of functional modules using network topology and high-throughput data. *BMC Systems Biology*, **1**, 8.

Vapnik, V. (1995). *The Nature of Statistical Learning Theory*. Springer, New York.

Yi, M., Horton, J. D., Cohen, J. C., Hobbs, H. H., and Stephens, R. M. (2006). WholePathwayScope: a comprehensive pathway-based analysis tool for high-throughput data. *BMC Bioinformatics* 2006, **7**, 30.

Yi, M., and Stephens, R. M. Seeking the unique and common biological themes in multiple gene lists or high-throughput datasets: high-throughput Pathway Pattern Extraction pipeline in WPS for pathway-level comparative analysis using pathway-level enrichment patterns and associated genes of patterned pathways. (Unpublished work)

Yi, M. and Stephens, R. M. (2008). SLEPR: A sample-level enrichment-based pathway ranking method – seeking biological themes through pathway-level consistency. *PLoS ONE*, **3(9)**, e3288.

Zanzoni, A., Montecchi-Palazzi, L., Quondam, M., Ausiello, G., Helmer-Citterich, M., and Cesareni, G. MINT: a Molecular INTeraction database. *FEBS Lett* 2002, **513**, 135–140.

Zeeberg, B. R., Feng, W., Wang, G., Wang, M. D., Fojo, A. T., Sunshine, M., Narasimhan, S., Kane, D. W., Reinhold, W. C., Lababidi, S., Bussey, K. J., Riss, J., J. Barrett C., and Weinstein, J. N. (2003). GoMiner: a resource for biological interpretation of genomic and proteomic data. *Genome Biology*, **4**, R28.

7

TWO METHODS FOR COMPARING GENOMIC DATA ACROSS INDEPENDENT STUDIES IN CANCER RESEARCH: META-ANALYSIS AND ONCOMINE CONCEPTS MAP

Wendy Lockwood Banka, Matthew J. Anstett and Daniel R. Rhodes

7.1 Introduction

Microarray experiments measure thousands of genes in every biological sample examined, and produce far richer result sets than conventional experimental approaches. The Oncomine project began in 2002 with the recognition that published genomic profiling data has a high latent value that can be exploited by assembling existing microarray data into a single, standardized database, linking the data with a sophisticated set of analysis tools, and making the resource available through a web-based interface (Rhodes et al., 2004a). By mid-2007 the Oncomine database and application contained over 500 million data points from 310 human oncology studies, a suite of analysis tools specifically designed for biologists, and a large user group that includes nearly 5000 cancer researchers worldwide. Oncomine is freely available to academic researchers at www.oncomine.org.

Oncomine contains gene expression data on tens of thousands of genes in thousands of samples that include normal tissues, diseased tissues, and cell lines, making it a powerful resource for discovering the expression patterns of individual genes. In addition, basic statistical analyses are run on every study that assembles genes on the basis of similar expression patterns between genes (co-expression), or on differences in expression between samples (differential expression) (Rhodes et al., 2007a). Oncomine also implements a novel statistical technique called Cancer Outlier Profile Analysis (COPA), which aims to identify significant over-expression that occurs in only a subset of samples (Tomlins et al., 2005).

Here we focus on two methods that go beyond analyses of individual genes or studies, and that instead attempt to capitalize on the coexistence of multiple standardized data sets within a single database. Meta-analysis compares the differential expression results calculated by Oncomine across studies, allowing researchers to distinguish between genes with robust expression from those that are less reliable. In contrast, Oncomine Concepts Map (OCM) is a database and application that compares a large and growing collection of gene lists derived from a variety of sources (Rhodes et al., 2007b; Tomlins et al., 2007). Users can interrogate concepts of interest using any of the 33,000+ gene lists already present, or can upload their own lists to compare against the collection. While OCM can be used for the same type of validation generated by meta-analysis, it is more widely used as a tool for expanding results from one experiment to those of another, with the goal of understanding the complex interactions between tumours, pathways, drugs, and biology.

7.2 Single-study gene expression analyses in Oncomine

Individual data sets are downloaded from public web sites such as GEO (Barrett et al., 2007), ArrayExpress (Parkinson et al., 2007), or the Stanford Microarray Database (Demeter et al., 2007), or are provided by authors upon request. Expression data are provided as two-channel ratio data or single-channel intensity data, and are typically retrieved in single composite file format. All available data are included in processing and analysis, except for negative single-channel intensity values. All expression data sets are log transformed and median centred per array, and standard deviations are normalized to one per array (Rhodes et al., 2007a).

Comparing results across studies using different array technologies requires that the language of individual array types (reporter IDs) be translated into a language that is common between them (genes). Reporter to gene mappings provided by commercial array manufacturers are not used since they are often out of date with respect to other public sources, such as UniGene and Entrez Gene. Instead, Reporter IDs are mapped directly to RefSeq or GenBank, and then to Entrez Gene using the following strategies:

- Reporter ID → RefSeq → Entrez Gene Mapping
- Reporter ID → GenBank Accession → Entrez Gene Mapping
- Reporter ID → GenBank Accession → UniGene → Entrez Gene Mapping

Note that Entrez Gene provides direct mappings for most RefSeqs, but not to all GenBank mRNA and EST sequences. When possible, direct Entrez Gene mappings are used. For all remaining reporters it is determined whether the GenBank sequence has been clustered by UniGene, and if so, the UniGene → Entrez Gene mapping is applied.

7.2.1 Differential expression analysis

All multi-study analyses described here begin with the results of differential expression or co-expression analyses on individual studies. For differential expression analyses, each data set is reviewed for potential comparisons of interest, such as:

- cancer versus respective normal tissue;
- high grade (undifferentiated) cancer versus low grade (differentiated) cancer;
- poor outcome (metastases, recurrence, or cancer-specific death) versus good outcome (long-term or recurrence-free survival);
- metastasized versus primary cancer;
- subtype 1 versus subtype 2.

Samples are assigned to classes such that the most advanced or the most negative of the options is designated Class 2 (e.g. 'cancer'), whereas the reference option is Class 1 (e.g. 'normal'). This provides consistent directionality to the analyses, which is necessary when making cross-study comparisons. Once the samples are classified and designated for analysis, Oncomine calculates the mean expression of each gene in each class, and then determines the statistical significance of the difference using the Student's t test; t tests are conducted as two-sided for differential expression analysis, and one-sided for over- or under-expression analysis. To calculate the Q-value (or gene-specific false discovery rate), genes are sorted by P, and then the ratio of the expected number of occurrences at or better than each P to the actual number of occurrences is computed (Storey and Tibshirani, 2003):

$$\text{Q-value} = (pn)/i$$

where
$p = P$;
n = total number of genes (inferences);
i = index (number of genes at or better than P).

Study: Beer_Lung
Analysis: Lung - Type
Class 1: Normal Lung (10)
Class 2: Lung Adenocarinoma (86)
Measured: 6856   **Up:** 1043 (15.2%)   **Down:** 1274 (18.6%)   **Diff:** 2307 (33.6%)

(Over Expressed Gene List)

Rank	Gene Symbol	Reporter ID	Count 1	Count 2	Mean 1	Mean 2	T-test	P-Value	Q Value
1	PSMD11	AB003102_at	10	86	.536	.8677	-11.23	2.4E-18	1.7E-14
2	ILF2	U10323_at	10	86	.7929	1.1685	-12.96	3.4E-18	1.2E-14
3	PSMB2	D26599_at	10	86	1.2426	1.5934	-13.12	4.6E-18	1E-14
4	EIF3S9	U78525_at	10	85	.5381	.9904	-12.183	2.7E-16	4.7E-13
5	P4HB	X05130_s_at	10	86	1.3402	1.8236	-14.969	1.3E-13	1.8E-10
6	PYCR1	M77836_at	10	86	.3976	.9582	-11.707	1.6E-13	1.8E-10
7	NONO	U02493_at	10	86	1.4171	1.6702	-9.433	5.5E-13	5.4E-10
8	UBE2C	U73379_at	10	86	.2887	.9544	-10.232	1.1E-12	9.4E-10
9	DAP	X76105_at	10	86	.5275	.945	-9.916	1.2E-12	9.1E-10
10	C20orf24	S83364_at	10	86	.0728	.3836	-8.549	1.3E-12	9.1E-10

Study: Beer_Lung   **Analysis:** Lung - Type
Class 1: Normal Lung (10)
Class 2: Lung Adenocarinoma (86)
Measured: 6856   **Up:** 1043 (15.2%)   **Down:** 1274 (18.6%)   **Diff:** 2307 (33.6%)

Gene Symbol	Q value
PSMD11	1.7E-14
ILF2	1.2E-14
PSMB2	1E-14
EIF3B	4.7E-13
P4HB	1.8E-10
PYCR1	1.8E-10
NONO	5.4E-10
UBE2C	9.4E-10
DAP	9.1E-10

FIG. 7.1: Sample Differential Expression Gene List and Heat Map results from a single study (Beer_Lung) that compares gene expression in Lung Adenocarcinoma to Normal Lung in Oncomine. Genes are ranked by Q-value. See Plate 5.

Oncomine uses the *p*-value and Q-value to rank differential expression results in heat maps and gene lists throughout the application (Fig. 7.1). These values are also used to rank the results for individual genes across studies in meta-analyses, and to generate gene signatures in Oncomine Concepts Map, as discussed below.

7.2.2 Co-expression analysis

Co-expression analysis is used to identify groups of genes from large gene sets that have similar expression patterns that can, for example, indicate interactions between genes involved in a cancer pathway (Rhodes *et al.*, 2007a,b). This process begins with calculation of the variance of each gene across all samples in a study, and selection of the top 10,000 most variable genes. Standard average linkage hierarchical clustering is then used to identify significant clusters of co-expressed genes among the 10,000 most variable genes. Thus a Gene Search in Oncomine, followed by navigation to the 'co-ex' tab, retrieves a list of all studies for which the queried gene was one of the top 10,000 most variable genes and was also a member of a cluster of similarly expressed genes. Results for any individual study can be visualized as either a gene list or as a heat map, as shown in Fig. 7.2. Co-expression clusters are also used to generate concepts in Oncomine Concepts Map, as discussed below.

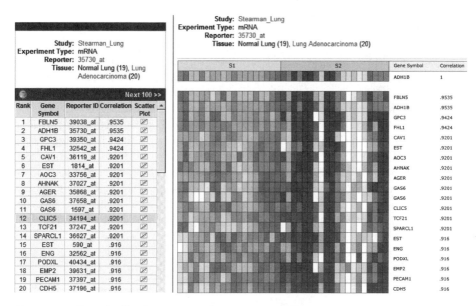

FIG. 7.2: Sample Co-Expression Gene List and Heat Map results from a single study (Stearman_Lung) containing Normal Lung and Lung Adenocarcinoma samples in Oncomine. The ADH1B cluster has a correlation of 0.9201 (correlation value of the 10th ranked gene) with a count size of 14 (number of genes that have a correlation of 0.9201 or better). See Plate 6.

7.3 Meta-analysis

Microarray technologies generate false positive results for a number of reasons, making it important to devise strategies for selecting only the most promising candidate genes for further research (reviewed in Rhodes and Chinnaiyan, 2004b). One obvious approach is to compare the results of different studies to determine which genes are differentially expressed repeatedly, across different labs and different microarray platforms. This solution is difficult to implement, however, because raw microarray data from different studies is generally not directly comparable (Kuo *et al.*, 2002; Tan *et al.*, 2003). An important breakthrough came with the observation that while experimental variability may cause expression levels of a gene to vary randomly between studies, the results of differential expression analyses for that gene – the difference in expression of a gene between normal and cancer tissues, for example – should be relatively constant (Rhodes *et al.*, 2002; Rhodes *et al.*, 2004c). In Oncomine, differential expression results for each gene are reported in statistical terms, as p-values and Q-values, as described above. The meta-analysis function builds on these calculations by comparing p-values in selected differential expression analyses from different studies, and reporting a list of genes ranked by p-values across these studies. As the size of the database has grown, so has the potential for using meta-analysis to make such cross-study comparisons (Niemantsverdreit *et al.*, 2007; Sharifi *et al.*, 2007; Wilson and Giguere, 2007).

7.4 Application

An example of an Oncomine meta-analysis is shown in Fig. 7.3. A Profile Search was used to identify all lung studies available in Oncomine, and then four identical analysis types (Class 1 = Normal; Class 2 = Lung Adenocarcinoma) from four independent studies (Garber *et al.*, 2001; Bhattacharjee *et al.*, 2001; Beer *et al.*, 2002; Stearman *et al.*, 2005), were selected for meta-analysis.

Meta-analysis results are visualized in two ways. The gene list view provides a ranked list showing the gene name, the list of studies in which that gene was over- or under-expressed, the p-value for that study, and a link to a box plot view of the data distribution. Alternatively, the Metamap view provides a view in which each study is a column and each gene a row, with the level of significant expression indicated by colour. This provides a visual cue of the level of over- (red) or under-expression (blue). The heat map also shows a single p-value, and a link to a box plot view of the underlying data.

For both the gene list and the Metamap visualizations, the method for ranking depends on the number of studies selected in the Study Count window. When Study Count = 1, Oncomine generates a list that is ranked by the most significant p-values across the selected studies, irrespective of overlap between studies. Note that in this case the p-value reported in the heat map corresponds to the most significant p-value reported in the four analyses (Fig. 7.3a). When Study Count = 2, Oncomine generates a list that is ranked by the second most significant p-value for each gene (Fig. 7.3b).

Application

(a)

Study Count: 1 — Under Expressed Gene List — Next 100 >>

Gene	Study	P-Value	Box Plot
ADH1B	Bhattacharjee_Lung	1.2E-16	View
	Garber_Lung	2.3E-7	
	Beer_Lung	5.1E-25	
	Stearman_Lung	1.3E-7	
CLEC3B	Bhattacharjee_Lung	2.2E-16	View
	Garber_Lung	6.2E-4	
	Beer_Lung	9.9E-25	
	Stearman_Lung	5.4E-11	
SEPP1	Bhattacharjee_Lung	1.6E-5	View
	Garber_Lung	0.007	
	Beer_Lung	1.3E-24	
	Stearman_Lung	2.9E-5	
NFE2L2	Bhattacharjee_Lung	0.464	View
	Garber_Lung	0.211	
	Beer_Lung	1.3E-22	
	Stearman_Lung	2.9E-5	
MEF2C	Bhattacharjee_Lung	0.068	View
	Garber_Lung	6.6E-4	
	Beer_Lung	1.3E-21	

1	2	3	4	Gene Symbol	P-Value (2)
				ADH1B	5.1E-25
				CLEC3B	9.92E-25
				SEPP1	1.35E-24
				NFE2L2	1.27E-22
				MEF2C	1.26E-21
				CYP4B1	1.96E-21
				FHL1	2.29E-20
				EMCN	1.09E-19
				FMO2	2.92E-19
				GPM6B	4.32E-19
				FEZ1	1.13E-18
				GPC3	4.17E-18
				CAV1	4.21E-18
				GMFG	4.43E-18
				SFTPA1B	6.3E-18
				HYAL2	8.31E-18
				MYLK	1.27E-17
				RAMP2	1.64E-17
				ADH1A	3.23E-17
				GRK5	3.89E-17

(b)

Study Count: 2 — Under Expressed Gene List — Next 100 >>

Gene	Study	P-Value	Box Plot
CAV1	Bhattacharjee_Lung	5.1E-11	View
	Garber_Lung	1.1E-17	
	Beer_Lung	4.2E-18	
	Stearman_Lung	9.3E-8	
ADH1B	Bhattacharjee_Lung	1.2E-16	View
	Garber_Lung	2.3E-7	
	Beer_Lung	5.1E-25	
	Stearman_Lung	1.3E-7	
CLEC3B	Bhattacharjee_Lung	2.2E-16	View
	Garber_Lung	6.2E-4	
	Beer_Lung	9.9E-25	
	Stearman_Lung	5.4E-11	
FHL1	Bhattacharjee_Lung	6E-16	View
	Garber_Lung	6.3E-10	
	Beer_Lung	2.3E-20	
	Stearman_Lung	1.5E-8	
GRK5	Bhattacharjee_Lung	3.9E-17	View
	Garber_Lung	1.2E-8	
	Beer_Lung	7.9E-11	

1	2	3	4	Gene Symbol	P-Value (2)
				CAV1	1.07E-17
				ADH1B	1.19E-16
				CLEC3B	2.21E-16
				FHL1	6.02E-16
				GRK5	7.32E-16
				AOC3	7.71E-15
				MYLK	2.24E-14
				VWF	1.46E-13
				RAMP2	1.63E-13
				AQP1	1.83E-13
				CDH5	2.59E-13
				HEG1	3.12E-13
				GPC3	4.95E-13
				ANGPT1	8.02E-13
				COX7A1	1.19E-12
				MYL9	1.2E-12
				SPOCK2	1.75E-12
				TEK	2.89E-12
				ADH1A	7.12E-12
				FEZ1	1.7E-11

FIG. 7.3: *Continued.*

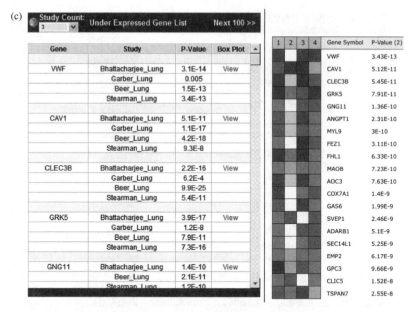

FIG. 7.3: Gene Lists and Heat Maps from Normal Lung vs. Lung Adenocarcinoma in four studies showing the effects of varying the Study Count. (a) For Study Count = 1, results are ranked by the most significant p-value for each gene. (b) For Study Count = 2, results are ranked by the second most significant p-value for each gene. (c) For Study Count = 3, results are ranked by the third most significant p-value for each gene. (d) For Study Count = 4, results are ranked by the fourth most significant p-value for each gene.

The advantage of using very strict criteria – in this example, Study Count = 4 generates a list ranked by the least significant p-value for each gene across the four studies (Fig. 7.3d) – is that the resulting list is highly conservative, and the results very likely to be real. The disadvantage is that this is likely an underrepresentation of relevant genes, since genes that are not measured on every platform, or that are poorly measured in a single case will not rank. For these reasons many users utilize the default 'leave-one-out' strategy of selecting a Study Count that is one less than the total number of studies compared (Fig. 7.3c).

7.5 Oncomine Concepts Map

An alternative approach for comparing results across studies is Oncomine Concepts Map (OCM) (Rhodes et al., 2007b; Tomlins et al., 2007). Like meta-analysis, this method often begins with the results of single study differential expression analysis in Oncomine. However, while meta-analysis compares p-values of individual genes, OCM compares the overlap of sets of genes – often referred to as gene signatures – between different experiments.

7.5.1 Assembling gene signatures

Oncomine Concepts Map is similar in structure to Oncomine in that it is a combination of data repository, analysis tools, and web-based user interface. However, instead of using microarray data as its source, OCM is built around a large and growing repository of gene signatures. Many of these signatures are derived from differential and co-expression analyses in Oncomine, which in OCM are called Oncomine Gene Expression Signatures and Oncomine Cluster Signatures, respectively. Other lists are manually curated from the literature, or are downloaded from public sources. A full list of concepts currently available in OCM is shown in Table 7.1.

Here we focus on the two types of concepts that are generated directly from the Oncomine database. First, for every differential expression analysis conducted in Oncomine, six Oncomine Concept lists are generated:

- Top 1 % Over-Expressed in Class 2 vs. Class 1
- Top 5 % Over-Expressed in Class 2 vs. Class 1
- Top 10 % Over-Expressed in Class 2 vs. Class 1
- Top 1 % Under-Expressed in Class 2 vs. Class 1
- Top 5 % Under-Expressed in Class 2 vs. Class 1
- Top 10 % Under-Expressed in Class 2 vs. Class 1

Thus for each of the four Lung Adenocarcinoma vs. Normal Lung analyses described in the Oncomine meta-analysis example, Oncomine Concepts Map contains six gene signatures representing different percentages of over- and under-expressed genes that resulted from those comparisons.

In addition to generating concepts based on differential expression analysis, OCM generates and stores an additional set of concepts, called Oncomine

TABLE 7.1. Source and number of gene signatures available in Oncomine Concepts Map.

OCM Concept Types	Number
• Oncomine Gene Expression Signatures	10,522
• Oncomine Cluster Signatures	11,166
• Literature-defined Concepts	657
• HPRD Interaction Sets	4144
• InterPro Protein Domains and Families	2072
• Connectivity Map Drug Signatures	1516
• GO Biological Process	855
• GO Cellular Component	249
• GO Molecular Function	818
• Transfac Transcription Factor Targets	361
• Chromosome Cytoband	314
• Biocarta Pathway	260
• Conserved Promoter Motifs	174
• picTar predicted miRNA target genes	168
• KEGG Pathway	160
• Conserved UTR Motifs	72
• PINdb Nuclear Protein Complexes	65
• Chromosome Arm	48
TOTAL	**33,621**

Cluster Signatures, that are derived from the results of co-expression analyses: co-expression clusters with 20 or more reporters with correlation of 0.5 or higher are added as individual gene lists to Oncomine Concepts Map. Because some reporters map to the same gene (or to no gene), actual gene cluster sizes in OCM may be smaller. For the four lung adenocarcinoma studies described above, OCM generated the 55 Oncomine Cluster Concepts shown in Table 7.2.

7.5.2 *Association analysis*

In addition to acting as a repository for individual gene signatures, Oncomine Concepts Map conducts large-scale association analysis across all concepts in the database. Molecular concepts are stored in a relational database schema that stratifies concepts by type, and that associates genes with Entrez Gene identifiers. In addition, each concept is assigned a 'null set', which represents the full set of genes from which the concept genes were defined. Every possible pair of concepts is tested for significant overlap by counting the number of genes

TABLE 7.2. Summary of the number and sizes of Oncomine Cluster Signatures derived from co-expression analyses of four different lung studies in Oncomine.

Study Name	Number of Clusters	Size of Largest Cluster	Size of Smallest Cluster
Beer_Lung	3	29 genes	23 genes
Bhattacharjee_Lung	14	296 genes	13 genes
Garber_Lung	28	162 genes	6 genes
Stearman_Lung	10	323 genes	16 genes

measured and present in both concepts, and assessing the significance of overlap using Fisher's exact test. Results are stored if a given test has an Odds Ratio greater than 1.25 and a p-value less than 0.01. p-values less than 1e-100 are set to 1e-100 (Rhodes et al., 2007b).

The Oncomine Concepts Map web interface also allows users to upload concepts privately. Each of these additional gene lists is compared in the same way to each of the other 33,000+ public concepts available in OCM, but the results are only viewable by that particular user.

7.6 Application

7.6.1 *Direct comparison of Oncomine concepts results to meta-analysis results*

Since differential expression analyses are the basis both for the individual signatures compared in meta-analysis, and for the gene signature concepts stored in Oncomine Concepts Map, it is possible to use Oncomine Concepts Map as an alternative to meta-analysis for directly comparing gene lists from different studies. For example, data from the same four lung adenocarcinoma studies used in the previous example can also be identified by doing a Concept Search on 'lung adenocarcinoma' in Oncomine Concepts Map, followed by selection of Concept: Lung Type – 'Top 10% under-expressed in Lung Adenocarcinoma (Garber)'. This concept can be used as a query concept to find similar signatures, using filters to focus on 'lung' and 'cancer vs. normal' (Fig. 7.4).

Once identified, concepts of interest can be selected, and comparisons between gene lists visualized as a network, heat map (overlay), or table. Not surprisingly, a direct comparison of the gene list derived from Oncomine Concepts Map closely matches the one derived from meta-analysis in this example where the exact same analyses were used as the starting point (data not shown); the size of the resulting gene lists and degree of overlap depends on the criteria used in each. However, while a set of validated, overlapping genes is generally the end-point in meta-analysis, in Oncomine Concepts Map it is the starting point for a series of additional queries.

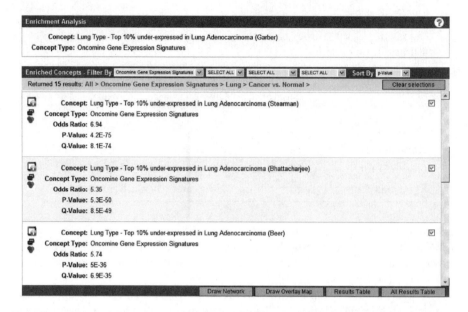

FIG. 7.4: Normal Lung vs. Lung Adenocarcinoma concepts in OCM corresponding to the same four analyses used in the meta-analysis in Fig. 7.3.

To demonstrate how this is accomplished, the gene list derived from the meta-analysis example (Fig. 7.3d) was uploaded into Oncomine Concepts Map. During Concept Upload, Oncomine automatically computed the association of the new gene list with the 33,000+ concepts already in the database, and then provided an interface for exploring the results. The meta-lung adenocarcinoma list was significantly associated with 1959 existing concepts in OCM, providing many opportunities for exploring relationships between genes on this list and those involved in a range of other biological processes.

One basic question that can be asked is where the genes on the list are expressed in normal tissue: one concept showing significant interaction with the meta-lung query concept is Yanai_Normal (Yanai et al., 2005). Selecting the analysis button associated with this concept retrieves a heat-map of genes differentially expressed between lung and a variety of other normal tissues, filtered by the genes from our meta-lung query concept. That is, only genes from the Yanai analysis (genes over-expressed in lung compared to other normal tissues) that are also in the meta-lung concept are shown (Fig. 7.5). Note that this result immediately shows that a number of genes that are under-expressed in lung adenocarcinoma (the query concept) are significantly over-expressed in normal lung when compared to other normal tissues.

It may also be of interest to know if other cancer types, when compared to their normal counterpart, similarly under-express the set of genes identified in the meta-analysis of lung adenocarcinoma example. Results from Fig. 7.6 show

Application

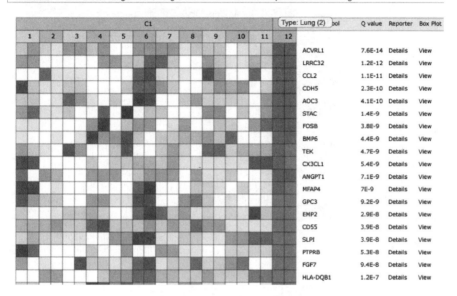

FIG. 7.5: Heat map of genes over-expressed in normal lung as compared to a number of other normal tissues, filtered by the set of genes identified in a meta-analysis of genes under-expressed in lung adenocarcinoma as compared to normal lung. See Plate 7.

that both prostate (Welsh et al., 2001) and ovary (Lu et al., 2004) cancers show similar under-expression when compared to normal tissues.

In addition to measuring the association of the query concept against other Oncomine gene signatures, Oncomine Concepts Map contains a wide range of biological concepts derived from other sources (Table 7.1). Filtering on Concepts within the KEGG pathway, for example, shows that genes on the meta-lung adenocarcinoma list significantly overlap with genes involved in the regulation of the actin cytoskeleton, the coagulation cascade, and other biochemical pathways (Fig. 7.7a). Similarly, by searching on Concepts within the Transfac Transcription Factor Targets, it is possible to identify transcription factors that associate significantly with this concept (Fig 7.7b). These results show how comparing the gene list from one experiment to gene lists derived from other experiments can provide unexpected insights and open new lines of inquiry. Beginning this type of open-ended inquiry with a highly validated meta-analysis signature, as shown here, is likely to be an effective strategy for ensuring that the query concept contains genes with a high likelihood of real biological significance.

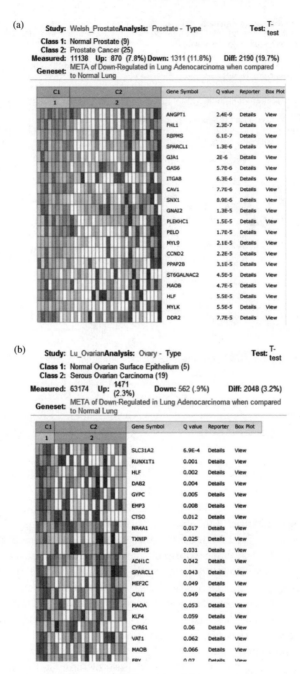

FIG. 7.6: Heat map of genes under-expressed in cancer as compared to normal tissues, filtered by the set of genes identified in a meta-analysis of genes under-expressed in lung adenocarcinoma as compared to normal lung. (a) Normal prostate vs. prostate cancer. (b) Normal ovary vs. ovarian carcinoma. See Plate 8.

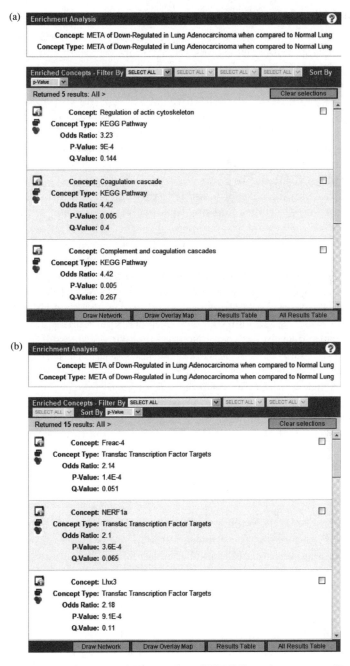

FIG. 7.7: Oncomine Concepts Map results of KEGG pathway genes lists (a) and Transfac Transcription Targets (b) that associate with genes identified in a meta-analysis of genes under-expressed in lung adenocarcinoma as compared to normal lung.

7.7 Conclusion

In summary, we have demonstrated two methods by which Oncomine re-utilizes data from multiple published studies to drive further insight into existing data and to advance cancer research.

Meta-analysis of microarrays relies on the comparison of gene expression between two classes of samples within the study – in our example normal lung vs. lung adenocarcinoma – as a reliable measure that can be used to compare results across studies, in a way that raw expression values from a single class of samples (lung adenocarcinoma) cannot. Oncomine automatically calculates these differential expression values for every gene in selected comparison types, and makes them available to users for a variety of purposes including meta-analysis. Meta-analysis makes it possible to distinguish and focus on results that are consistent across studies and are thus likely to represent actual biological events.

Oncomine Concepts Map begins with data from the same differential expression analyses, but stores the results as gene lists encompassing the top 1, 5, and 10 % of genes that are over- or under-expressed in each analysis. While these gene lists can be used, as in meta-analysis, to validate results across studies, the real value of OCM is that it provides a systematic way to compare gene lists derived from a variety of sources, opening new opportunities for assessing the degree of genetic overlap between disparate biological processes.

Importantly, none of the individual methods described here involve highly complicated statistical analysis techniques. Rather, the impact of this effort relies on the continued accumulation of large quantities of existing data, curation to provide complete and accurate datas ets, organization of the data into a standard format, and the development of an intuitive interface. To date Oncomine has facilitated many novel discoveries that have contributed to the biological understanding of cancer, as well as to the broader effort of diagnosing and treating this complex disease.

References

Barrett, T., Troup, D. B., Wilhite, S. E., Ledoux, P., Rudnev, D., Evangelista, C., Kim, I. F., Soboleva, A., Tomashevsky, M., and Edgar, R. (2007). NCBI GEO: mining tens of millions of expression profiles – database and tools update, *Nucleic Acids Res.*, 35, pp. D760–D5.

Beer, D. G., Kardia, S. L., Huang, C. C., Giordano, T. J., Levin, A. M., Misek, D. E., Lin, L., Chen, G., Gharib, T. G., Thomas, D. G., Lizyness, M. L., Kuick, R., Hayasaka, S., Taylor, J. M., Iannettoni, M. D., Orringer, M. B., and Hanash, S. (2002). Gene-expression profiles predict survival of patients with lung adenocarcinoma, *Nat. Med.*, 8, pp. 816–24.

Bhattacharjee, A., Richards, W. G., Staunton, J., Li, C., Monti, S., Vasa, P., Ladd, C., Beheshti, J., Bueno, R., Gillette, M., Loda, M., Weber, G., Mark, E. J., Lander, E. S., Wong, W., Johnson, B. E., Golub, T. R., Sugarbaker, D. J., and Meyerson, M. (2001). Classification of human lung carcinomas by mRNA expression profiling reveals distinct adenocarcinoma subclasses, *Proc. Natl. Acad. Sci. USA*, 98, pp. 13790–5.

Demeter, J., Beauheim, C., Gollub, J., Hernandez-Boussard, T., Jin, H., Maier, D., Matese, J., Nitzberg, M., Wymore, F., Zachariah, Z. K., Brown, P.O., Sherlock, G., and Ball, C. A. (2007). The Stanford Microarray Database: implementation of new analysis tools and open source release of software, *Nucleic Acids Res.*, 35, pp. D766–D70.

Garber, M. E., Troyanskaya, O. G., Schluens, K., Petersen, S., Thaesler, Z., Pacyna-Gengelbach, M., van de Rijn, M., Rosen, G. D., Perou, C. M., Whyte, R. I., Altman, R. B., Brown, P. O., Botstein, D., and Petersen, I., (2001). Diversity of gene expression in adenocarcinoma of the lung, *Proc. Natl. Acad. Sci. USA*, 98, pp. 13784–9.

Kuo, W. P., Jenssen, T. K., Butte, A. J., Ohno-Machado, L., and Kohane, I. S. (2002). Analysis of matched mRNA measurements from two different microarray technologies, *Bioinformatics*, 18, pp. 405–12.

Lu, K. H., Patterson, A. P., Wang, L., Marquez, R. T., Atkinson, E. N., Baggerly, K. A., Ramoth, L. R., Rosen, D. G., Liu, J., Hellstrom, I., Smith, D., Hartmann, L., Fishman, D., Berchuck, A., Schmandt, R., Whitaker, R., Gershenson, D. M., Mills, G. B., and Bast, R. C., Jr. (2004). Selection of potential markers for epithelial ovarian cancer with gene expression arrays and recursive descent partition analysis, *Clin. Cancer. Res.*, 10, pp. 3291–300.

Niemantsverdriet, M. Wagner, K., Visser, M., and Backendorf, C. (2008). Cellular functions of 14-3-3zeta in apoptosis and cell adhesion emphasize its oncogenic character, *Oncogene*, 20, pp. 1315–9.

Parkinson, H., Kapushesky, M., Shojatalab, M., Abeygunawardena, N., Coulson, R., Farne, A., Holloway, E., Kolesnykov, P., Lilja, P., Lukk, M., Mani, R., Rayner, T., Sharma, A., William, E., Sarkans, U., and Brazma, A. (2007). ArrayExpress – a public database of microarray experiments and gene expression profiles, *Nucleic Acids Res.*, 35, pp. D747–D50.

Rhodes, D. R., Barrette, T. R., Rubin, M. A., Ghosh, D., and Chinnaiyan, A. M. (2002). Meta-analysis of microarrays: interstudy validation of gene expression profiles reveals pathway dysregulation in prostate cancer, *Cancer Res.*, 62, pp. 4427–33.

Rhodes, D. R., Yu, J., Shanker, K., Deshpande, N., Varambally, R., Ghosh, D., Barrette, T., Pandey, A., and Chinnaiyan, A. M. (2004a). ONCOMINE: a cancer microarray database and integrated data-mining platform', *Neoplasia*, 6, pp. 1–6.

Rhodes, D. R. and Chinnaiyan, A. M. (2004b). Bioinformatics Strategies for Translating Genome-Wide Analyses into Clinically Useful Cancer Markers, *Ann. N. Y. Acad. Sci.*, pp. 32–40.

Rhodes, D. R., Yu, J., Shanker, K., Deshpande, N., Varambally, R., Ghosh, D., Barrette, T., Pandey, A., and Chinnaiyan, A. M. (2004c). Large-scale meta-analysis of cancer microarray data identifies common transcriptional profiles of neoplastic transformation and progression, *Proc. Natl. Acad. Sci. USA*, 101, pp. 9309–14.

Rhodes, D. R., Kalyana-Sundaram, S., Mahavisno, V., Varambally, R., Yu, J., Briggs, B. B., Barrette, T. R., Anstett, M.J., Kincaid-Beal, Kulkarni, P., Varambally, S., Ghosh, D., and Chinnaiyan, A. M. (2007a). Oncomine 3.0: genes, pathways, and networks in a collection of 18,000 cancer gene expression profiles, *Neoplasia*, 9, pp. 166–80.

Rhodes, D. R., Kalyana-Sundaram, S., Tomlins, S. A., Mahavisno, V., Kasper, N., Varambally, R., Barrette, T. R., Ghosh, D., Varambally, S., and Chinnaiyan, A. M. (2007b). Molecular concepts analysis links tumors, pathways, mechanisms, and drugs, *Neoplasia*, 9, pp. 443–54.

Sharifi, N., Hurt, E. M., Kawasaki, B. T., and Farrar, W. L. (2007). TGFBR3 loss and consequences in prostate cancer, *Prostate*, 67, pp. 301–11.

Stearman, R. S., Dwyer-Nield, L., Zerbe, L., Blaine, S. A., Chan, Z., Bunn, P. A., Jr., Johnson, G. L., Hirsch, F. R., Merrick, D. T., Franklin, W. A., Baron, A. E., Keith, R. L., Nemenoff, R. A., Malkinson, A. M., and Geraci, M. W. (2005). Analysis of orthologous gene expression between human pulmonary adenocarcinoma and a carcinogen-induced murine model, *Am. J. Pathol.*, 167, pp. 1763–75.

Storey, J. D. and Tibshirani, R. (2003). Statistical significance for genomewide studies, *Proc. Natl. Acad. Sci. USA*, 100, pp. 9440–5.

Tan, P. K., Downey, T. J., Spitznagel, E. L., Jr., Xu, P., Fu, D., and Dimitrov, D. S. (2003). Evaluation of gene expression measurements from commercial microarray platforms, *Nucleic Acids Res.*, 31, pp. 5676–84.

Tomlins, S. A., Mehra, R., Rhodes, D. R., Cao, X., Wang, L., Dhanasekaran, S. M., Kalyana-Sundaram, S., Wei, J. T., Rubin, M. A., Pienta, K. J., Shah, R. B., and Chinnaiyan, A. M. (2007). Integrative molecular concept modeling of prostate cancer progression, *Nat Genet*, 39, pp. 41–51.

Tomlins, S. A., Rhodes, D. R., Perner, S., Dhanasekaran, S. M., Mehra, R., Sun, X. W., Varambally, S., Cao, X., Tchinda, J., Kuefer, R., Lee, C., Montie, J. E., Shah, R. B., Pienta, K. J., Rubin, M. A. and Chinnaiyan, A. M. (2005). Recurrent fusion of TMPRSS2 and ETS transcription factor genes in prostate cancer, *Science*, 310, pp. 644–8.

Welsh, J. B., Sapinoso, L. M., Su, A. I., Kern, S. G., Wang-Rodriguez, J., Moskaluk, C. A., Frierson, H. F., Jr., and Hampton, G. M. (2001). Analysis of gene expression identifies candidate markers and pharmacological targets in prostate cancer, *Cancer Res.*, 61, pp. 5974–8.

Wilson, B. J. and Giguere, V. (2007). Identification of novel pathway partners of p68 and p72 RNA helicases through Oncomine meta-analysis, *BMC Genomics*, 8, p. 419.

Yanai, I., Benjamin, H., Shmoish, M., Chalifa-Caspi, V., Shklar, M., Ophir, R., Bar-Even, A., Horn-Saban, S., Safran, M., Domany, E., Lancet, D., and Shmueli, O. (2005). Genome-wide midrange transcription profiles reveal expression level relationships in human tissue specification, *Bioinformatics*, 21, pp. 650–9.

8

BIOINFORMATIC APPROACHES TO THE ANALYSIS OF ALTERNATIVE SPLICING VARIANTS IN CANCER BIOLOGY

Lue Ping Zhao, Jessica Andriesen and Wenhong Fan

8.1 Introduction to alternative splicing

Human genes, like those of other eukaryotes, contain intervening sequences that are present in the genomic DNA and are transcribed by transcription complexes, but do not get translated into the final protein product. These intervening sequences, termed introns, must get removed as part of the maturation process of the messenger RNA (mRNA) so that they do not become part of the translated message. The transcribed regions of the sequence that remain in the mature message are termed exons. The exonic sequences, together with the poly(A) tail, constitute the nucleic acids present in the mature mRNA.

The removal of introns from the pre-mRNA ocurrs by a process known as splicing. In general terms, the cellular splicing machinery (the spliceosome) catalyses the intramolecular joining of exon sequences in a sequence-specific way to produce a mature message. Consensus sequences that define the location of this joining, termed splice sites, play a major role in the determination of the resulting product. Much work has been done to identify the cellular components that make up the spliceosome and the sequences it recognizes, and so constitutive splicing is fairly well understood at the molecular level. However, throughout the quest to understand splicing at an overall level, other *cis*- and *trans*-elements that affect specific splice sites have been identified, implying a higher-order regulation of splicing and the existence of alternate splice forms which contribute to the diversity of cellular functions.

8.1.1 *Traditional methods for splicing analysis*

Traditional genetic systems were initially utilized to shed light on the mechanisms and understanding of constitutive as well as alternative splicing. Sex determination in *Drosophila melanogaster*, for example, was one of the initial systems used to understand splicing regulation and demonstrate that much of the same machinery is utilized for both systems (Hodges and Bernstein, 1994). In this system, as well as others, alternatively spliced genes were studied on a gene-by-gene basis, with the limitations of the molecular techniques available at the time. For example, Northern blots with exon-specific probes were often used to demonstrate the presence or absence of specific exons in transcripts of genes thought to undergo alternative splicing, such as the proto-oncogene *Sint1* (Sorensen *et al.*, 2002).

The use of the enzyme reverse transcriptase (RT) to generate cDNA from mRNA species opened up a new field of mRNA analysis. The combination of RT and polymerase chain reaction (PCR) gave scientists a way of amplifying and cloning even rare mRNA variants that could then be used for further studies. Large libraries of expressed sequence tags (ESTs) were generated from many tissues, species and timepoints in development. From these EST clones, longer-length cDNAs were identified, giving researchers their first glimpse at the world of alternatively spliced mRNA. Various types of alternative splicing were seen, including exon-skipping, alternatively used exons, the use of cryptic splice sites, the inclusion of so-called intronic sequences, and more (Fig. 8.1). However, these analyses were plagued with problems such as incomplete cDNA synthesis and encountered obstacles in the identification, annotation, and curation of such a large number of sequences (Matsubara and Okubo, 1993).

As illustrated here, alternative splice variants can arise from any combinations of exons or alternative exons. One theoretical question is how many different alternative splice variants can exist from a given number of exons. To proceed with a theoretical calculation, let us assume that a gene has N exons. Further, we assume that each exon can take three possible states: complete absence, presence of the entire exon, and partial presence. Under the assumption that each mature message must include the first and last exons, the total number of theoretical alternative splice variants equals 3^{N-2}. In addition, intronic sequence(s) may or may not be inserted into the mature message, resulting in another multiplier of 2^{N-1}. Collectively, the theoretical number of alternative splice variants can be

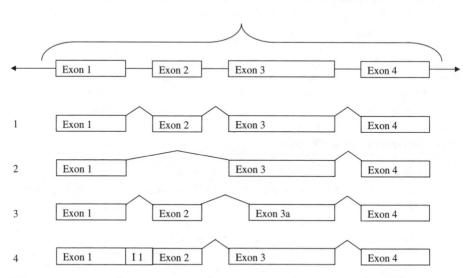

FIG. 8.1: Exemplified alternative splice variants within a hypothetical gene: (1) all exons are included; (2) exon skipping; (3) use of cryptic splice site generates an alternative exon 3 (exon 3a); (4) inclusion of intronic sequence in mature message.

as large as $2 \cdot 6^{N-2}$. When the number of exons within a gene is larger than five, the total number of variants can be quite substantial.

8.1.2 Current estimates of alternative splicing in humans

The number of known splice variants that occur in humans (the alternative transcriptome) is continually increasing. At present, over half of human genes have documented alternative splice forms, and several database repositories for annotating and curating these alternatively spliced sequences are currently maintained. For example, the Alternative Splicing and Transcript Diversity (ASTD) database project is run by the European Bioinformatics Institute. The ASAP II Database, which can be queried for cancer-specific alternative splice forms, is maintained by the University of California Los Angeles Bioinformatics Department, and both alternative and traditional splicing variants are collected in AceView from the National Center for Biotechnology Information (USA). These databases also contain information on alternative splicing in a number of additional species, including mouse, rat, nematodes, and others.

8.1.3 Alternative splicing and cancer

Although alternative splicing occurs commonly in normal cells and tissues, alterations of this process in cancer cells can result in the creation of new mRNA species or the alteration of ratios between isoforms in tissue-specific ways. There are numerous studies of specific genes with splicing alterations related to cancer (reviewed in Venables 2006); however, at this time it is still unclear whether these alterations are related to cancer biology or are merely by-products of pathways activated during the progression to disease. Nonetheless, this group of genes includes many well-known players including p53, TERT, and members of the caspase and Bcl2 families. Alternative splice forms have also been found in cancers of all stages. Thus, the questions for the study of alternative splicing as it relates to cancer biology are many-fold: how does alternative splicing evolve during this process? What is the role of alternatively spliced forms in the progression to cancer? Will limiting the splicing of these alternative forms slow disease progression? Can these patterns be used as biomarkers to detect and potentially treat certain cancer forms in a more effective way? Researchers aim to understand the types of changes that occur when cells become cancerous. However, single-gene specific analyses will not be sufficient to answer these questions, and cancer researchers have become reliant on large data sets primarily generated using oligonucleotide microarray technology.

8.2 Oligonucleotide arrays for detecting alternative splicing variants

The development of oligonucleotide microarray technology gave scientists a powerful tool for the analysis of alternative splicing. Currently, experiments that previously took years of library construction, sequence analysis and extensive annotation can be accomplished within a few months' time, with far fewer resources and smaller amounts of precious sample materials required. The types of microarrays utilized and their advantages and disadvantages for the study of alternative splicing are outlined below.

8.2.1 cDNA arrays

A typical cDNA array includes a large number of long probes that are complementary to the target sequences within candidate genes (Brown and Hartwell, 1998; Brown and Botstein, 1999). When test and reference samples labelled with two different fluorescent dyes are placed onto the array, the differential hybrizations of test and reference samples with probes are directly observed via measuring intensity values of the two dyes. Although this technology is primarily designed to study gene expression, it can be used for assessing alternative splicing variation when multiple probes are used to cover a single gene. However, this application has several limitations. The primary limitation is that cDNA arrays are typically constructed with relatively long, single probes for each gene. While this is adequate for assessing expression levels of transcripts if the target sequence is not spliced out, such a probe is not sufficiently useful for assessing alternative splice variants, either because the single probe sequence is unable to detect exon variations or the probe is too long to identify missing exons. To address this issue, some investigators have put effort into the development of customized arrays to detect alternative splicing. However, these studies can be cost prohibitive, and these arrays are often designed in a study-specific manner. Some commercially available array systems are a step increased from the previous systems. At this point, these arrays are often designed with information derived from large sequence databases, some of which are known to be biased, including the enrichment of 3' sequences due to the methods of EST and cDNA construction. The need to overcome such biases has stimulated a dynamic development of commercialized oligonucleotide arrays specifically designed for the study of splicing events.

8.2.2 GeneChip arrays

One commonly used array system is the GeneChip, produced by Affymetrix Inc. (www.affymetrix.com). In contrast to the typical two colour cDNA system that uses a single long probe, the GeneChip system uses multiple pairs of perfect- and mismatch probes (the actual number of pairs varies according to the chip version). A perfect-match probe has a short oligo sequence with 25 nucleotides that are perfectly matching with the targeting sequence. The mismatch probe has the same probe sequence, except for one nucleotide that is mismatched with the target sequence. Typically, multiple probe pairs cover different segments of the target transcript, and tend to be biased towards the 3' end. When these probes cover different exons, they can be effectively used to detect the presence of alternative splice variants (ASV). However, since it is designed to assess gene expression levels, the GeneChip array has major limitations when it is applied to assessing ASV. For example, the short oligo-probes are chosen without respect to optimizing the detection capability of ASV. In fact, many probes are located towards the 3′ end of the target sequence, covering a small portion of the gene, and hence are inadequate for assessing ASV. Recognition of this and other limitations has stimulated the development of alternative technologies for assessing ASV, such as exon arrays.

8.2.3 GeneChip exon arrays

To focus on increasing the detection capability of exons within each gene, Affymetrix Inc. has developed an exon array; the exon array uses one or more probes to cover each individual exon within each gene. Naturally, this technology is much more appropriate for assessing ASV throughout the genome. These arrays contain probes targeted specifically at exons, often with multiple probes per exon, enabling evaluation of expression at exon-specific as well as gene-specific levels. Because the probes are not based solely on pre-existing mRNA species, these arrays also facilitate the detection of novel splice forms.

Although this is a marked improvement over the use of GeneChip expression arrays from the perspective of assessing ASV, the content of these arrays is still not comprehensive. For example, the use of a cryptic splice site within an exon may result in the inclusion or exclusion of a large portion of the exon, giving a false read from an exon chip. Alternatively, the inclusion of 'intronic' sequences in the final RNA product may be missed, as these sequences may not be represented on the chip. Finally, the expression of unknown or unpredicted genes would not be accessible using this system. Overcoming these limitations motivated the development of tiling arrays (see below).

8.2.4 Tiling arrays

Perhaps the most robust and thorough evaluation of genomic sequence for RNA splicing comes from the use of genome tiling arrays. These arrays, in which oligonucleotide probes are based on sequences that are evenly spaced throughout the genome, are not limited to annotated genes and make no *a priori* assumptions about gene structure. These probes can either be partially overlapping or non-overlapping in nature. Preliminary studies using arrays of this type have generated evidence that much more of the genome is transcribed than originally thought (reviewed in Mockler *et al.*, 2005).

Tiling arrays have also been utilized as a mechanism for resequencing regions of the genome from many individual samples. In this case, the probes are tiled at a one base resolution, enabling the analysis of each nucleotide within the defined region. Information gathered from these analyses could help contribute to the study of alternative splicing by identifying functional polymorphisms that can then be correlated with known splicing outcomes, providing a genetic basis for observed differences seen betweeen groups of samples. These larger and more complicated array systems, however, present greater problems in terms of data analysis. With extremely large numbers of data points per sample, and probe hybridization characteristics dependent on many factors, careful interpretation of signals from microarrays must be made a priority. Never before has the need for bioinformatics and computational approaches to biological data analysis been so great.

8.3 Bioinformatic approaches

8.3.1 Two group design

8.3.1.1 *Matched design* Recognizing the complexity of gene expression and its variations across different cellular populations, one often considers a matched study design. Specifically, the study may include a group of randomly selected cancer patients who have been diagnosed with a solid tumour. As such a tumour is surgically removed, it is common that a relatively sizable piece of tissue, including the solid tumour, is removed from the cancerous organ. The removed tissue includes the targeted tumour tissue as well as 'normal' looking tissues, i.e. adjacent normal tissues. To compute the differences in alternative splice variants (ASV) between tissues, let vectors Y_{i1} and Y_{i0} denote the intensity values of probes that are used to measure the abundance of the corresponding expression levels in tumour and normal tissues, where the subscript i is used to denote the ith patient. For such a design, the most effective quantification of ASV is via modelling the difference vector $Z_i = Y_{i1} - Y_{i0}$. How to model this difference vector will be discussed below.

There are pros and cons associated with this design. The primary advantage of this design is that it enables the extraction of ASV information from the difference. Since the difference eliminates subject-specific variations, the difference vector quantifies only differentially expressed signals between cancerous and normal tissues. Hence, the resulting information is less likely confounded by any subject-specific variations, such as age, gender, or ethnicity, provided that such variables do interact with ASV. Statistically speaking, the results from analysing such difference data tend to be robust. On the other hand, natural variations associated with the difference $Z_i = Y_{i1} - Y_{i0}$ are increased, and the increment is determined by the intra-correlation between cancerous and normal tissues. On one extreme, Y_{i1} and Y_{i0} are highly correlated due to shared subject-specific effects. If so, the difference eliminates such subject-specific effects, without significantly increasing the variation. On the other extreme, variations in ASV assessments Y_{i1} and Y_{i0} are independent, and hence there is no need to control subject-specific effects. In this case, the variance of the difference could be doubled. If this is the case, it is much preferred to consider the unmatched design, described below.

8.3.1.2 *Unmatched design* In contrast to the matched design, an unmatched study design consists of collecting a random sample of cancerous tissues as the case samples, and a random sample of normal tissues as the control samples. Preferably, case and control samples are from different subjects, guaranteeing independence across all samples. Let the binary indicator $d_i = 1$ or 0 denote that the ith subject is a case or control, respectively. For modelling ASV, one would use an intensity value vector Y_{id_i} (with the additional index d_i) as the quantification of ASV information, i.e. $Z_{id_i} = Y_{id_i}$. The section below describes an analytic strategy for modelling such data.

Like the matched design, the unmatched design also has its strengths and weaknesses. The primary advantage is that this design is relatively easier to implement if normal biopsy samples are readily available. In addition, this design is potentially more efficient than the matched study design due to larger sample sizes for each of the two groups. However, this design becomes inferior to the matched design if the subject-to-subject variation is much greater than the subtle signals to be detected between cancerous and normal tissues.

8.3.2 Functional alternative splicing variants utilizing exon arrays

ASV may be an important mechanism for cells to produce sufficient diversity in their molecular repertoire. An earlier schematic (Fig 8.1) identifies the potential structure of multiple exons within a single gene. To enable the formalization of ASV analysis, we use a slightly different representation of the ASV data (Fig. 8.2). Suppose that a gene structure includes four exons with variable sizes. Within each exon, variable numbers of probe sets have been identified and incorporated into the oligonucleotide-array, indicated by small triangles. In the figure, the notation 'H' and 'L' is introduced to denote high and low expression

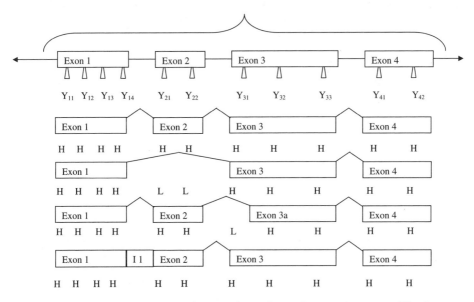

FIG. 8.2: Notation introduced for this hypothetical gene structure: Y_{kl} denotes the intensity value for the lth probe within the kth exon, and symbols H and L stand for relatively high or low intensity values for every probe. Indices i (subject) and j (gene) are suppressed here for convenience.

values, respectively, and thus, corresponding exons are detected with varying expression values. Now we use the subscript i for the ith subject, j for the jth gene, k for the kth exon, and l for the lth probe. Y_{ijkl} is used to denote the measurable signal for the corresponding probe. Suppose that for all possible ASV, the transcripts are configured to have exons 1 and 4, but exons 2 and 3 are alternatively spliced into four possible species: with or without exon 2, 3 or both. By expectation, numerical expression values for each probe set are relatively high if the corresponding exon is present, or are relatively low, otherwise.

While ASV are conceptually well-defined, detecting all possible ASV in a given biological sample is challenging. Presumably, a single gene could have multiple ASV within a single cell/tissue. Hence, actual measurements via oligo-arrays are average values of all ASV that contain the given probe sequence, thus the average values do not provide any information for ASV at the individual probe level.

Within the two group study, however, we are contrasting measurements between two groups probe-by-probe, and thus have an opportunity to detect differences of averaged measurements between two groups. Now if no difference is detected, one could conclude either that the targeted exon is not involved in the alternative splicing process, or that the target exon is involved in the alternative slicing process but the corresponding ASV is not associated with the cancerous development. On the other hand, if a statistically significant difference is detected, one would conclude not only the presence of ASV for the target exon, but also its association with the disease phenotype. Hence, we term such ASV as functional ASV hereafter.

8.3.3 A general framework

Consider an unmatched study with I independent subjects, who may be cases ($d_i = 1$) or controls ($d_i = 0$). The tissue sample from each subject is assayed with one of the array technologies described above. Suppose that each array includes J genes, with the subscript running from $j = 1$ to J. Each gene has variable numbers of exons, with the subscript $k = 1, 2, \ldots, K_j$. Further, each exon is covered by one or more probe sets, with l ranging from 1 to L_{jk}. For those exons not covered by any probe set, it is meaningless to incorporate such a variable. For each probe set, one typically has multiple probes, denoted by the subscript m. The actual number of probes is fixed depending on the choice of technology. For example, earlier versions of Affymetrix technology use 11 probe pairs, while recent versions use only four probes. Other oligonucleotide-array technology uses one single long probe. Now let Y_{ijklm} denote the intensity value for the jth gene, the kth exon, the lth probe set, and the mth probe in the ith subject. Here, another complexity, with Affymetrix technology in particular, is the use of a mismatch probe, and is ignored here, since it is no longer used in the newer chips. Aside from expression values, a study frequently collects one or more covariates x_i, such as age, gender, and medical history.

The intensity value, quantifying the abundance of the mRNA hybridized on a probe and denoted as Y_{ijklm}, is a random variable. Its average value is influenced by gene-specific, exon-specific, probe-specific hybridization, non-specific random hybridization on chip, and, finally, biological/sample-specific variations. To meaningfully capture biological variations, one would have to model multi-level sources of random variations. A linear model is typically desired, and may be written as

$$Y_{ijklm} = \delta_i + \lambda_i(\alpha_{jklm} + \beta_{jk}d_i) + \varepsilon_{ijklm}, \tag{8.1}$$

where α_{jklm} is associated with the probe-specific and non-specific hybridization, and β_{jk} quantifies the difference between cancerous and normal tissues for the kth exon within the jth gene while δ_i and λ_i are heterogeneous factors to be estimated. When array data are appropriately normalized, δ_i are around zero, and λ_i centres around 1. In general, introduction of both parameters ensures correction of heterogeneity prior to the final association analysis, a good analytic practice. The random residual ε_{ijklm} is assumed to be independent across subjects and may be correlated among multiple probes within the probe set, among multiple probes within the exon, and among multiple exons within the gene, except that the correlation structure is unspecified. Furthermore, its random distribution is unspecified.

Focusing on our primary analytic objective, which is to estimate α_{jklm} and β_{jk}, we have introduced an idea of applying an estimating equation technique (Fan et al., 2006). Basically, one can establish an estimating equation for estimating the mean parameters α_{jklm} and β_{jk} via modelling the marginal mean vector $\mu_i = (\mu_{11i}, \ldots, \mu_{jki}, \ldots)$, which may be written as $E(Y_i) = \{E(Y_{ijklm})\}$ given disease status. Generically, the estimating equation, with identity weight matrix, can be written as

$$\sum_{i=1}^{I} \frac{\partial \mu_i}{\partial (\underline{\alpha}, \underline{\beta})}(Y_i - \mu_i) = 0, \tag{8.2}$$

where $\underline{\alpha}$ and $\underline{\beta}$ are vectors of parameters specified in the above eqn (8.1). This estimating equation may not be considered statistically efficient, because all covariances between probes are set to zero, leading to an identity weight matrix. However, the construction of this estimating equation leads to a simplified and explicit expression for computation, hence leading to a computationally efficient implementation. It is easily scalable to process a large number of probes. As a general theory, the estimating equation technique was proposed in the early 1970s, and was made popular by Liang and Zeger (1986). The basic idea is that one can obtain a consistent estimate of parameters using moments, such as means, variances, and covariances, from an estimating equation, without requiring any distributional assumption. Its performance is expected to be more robust than the likelihood estimate, mostly because the former requires no distributional assumption, while the latter does. After obtaining consistent estimates, the estimating equation theorem (Liang and Zeger, 1986) will render an estimate of the covariance matrix for estimated parameters. Such a covariance matrix can be used for making statistical inference, when asymptotic theory is applicable.

For the matched design, the above framework is readily applicable with some modifications. The primary modification is that all probe intensity values need to be modified prior to taking their differences between cancerous and normal tissues. Some well-established algorithms for modification are implemented in RMA (Barash et al., 2004) or in GPM schema (Fan et al., 2006). Basically, one needs to adjust for unequal subject specific terms δ_i and λ_i, resulting in a modified intensity value $\widehat{Y}_i$. Following modification, one can compute the difference as $Z_i = \widehat{Y}_{i1} - \widehat{Y}_{i0}$, where the additional subscript 1 and 0 indicates case and control, respectively. To quantify ASV, one may use the following modified model as $Z_{ijklm} = \beta_{jk} + \varepsilon_{ijklm}$. Under such a model, the primary goal is to estimate β_{jk}, and to assess if β_{jk} is significantly greater or less than zero. Note that the intercept α_{jklm} is excluded, because it equals zero by the matching design. Again, the estimating equation technique is applicable for estimating a covariance matrix, which can be used for making inferences on parameters of interest. Specifically, the ratio of estimated coefficient over the estimate variance square-root, i.e. signal-to-noise ratio, is statistically known as the Z-score. Under the null hypothesis that the true coefficient equals zero, this Z-score would have a normal distribution. Hence, one can use this normal distribution to compute a p-value. With an appropriate account for multiple comparisons, one can set up a threshold value for significance based on the p-value. A significant result would indicate the presence of a functional ASV.

8.3.4 Relative versus absolute abundance

One important aspect in quantifying functional ASV is the choice of the measurement scale, i.e. using relative abundance or using absolute abundance. MIDAS by Affymetrix is software whose computational algorithm generally uses the same statistical framework as above, but quantifies ASV via relative abundance. Basically, MIDAS quantifies signal levels for each exon, and then computes the relative abundance of each exon over all exons within the gene. The relative abundance measurements are then used in all downstream analyses. In contrast, Partek® Genomics Suite, implemented by Partek, also uses virtually the same modelling framework as described above, except that it uses exon- and probe-specific intensity values as their absolute abundance measures.

While the statistical framework described here is applicable to either relative or absolute measurements, the choice of the scale hinges on the underlying assumptions about exon signals of interest. In the ideal situation, where signals for multiple exons within a gene are numerically comparable, the relative abundance measurements via ratios would be preferred, because this calculation normalizes exon-specific signals across multiple exons. Furthermore, its ratios are independent of the overall abundance of that gene. Hence, the ratio-based analysis will be more robust. On the other hand, calculated ratios in some exons may have an inflated variance due to variations associated with other exons. Consequently, the analysis may become less efficient.

By using absolute abundance, one implicitly assumes that the intensity values are directly indicative of ASV at various exons. When the normalization across chips and across exons is adequately performed, the normalized intensity value can be directly used for measuring the abundance of individual exons. Hence, such an analysis would be efficient and straightforward. However, this analysis may produce misleading results if probe-level normalization is inadequate.

More research is required to investigate pros and cons associated with each of these two choices, and future studies with alternate array types may reveal which technique gives more robust, accurate results.

8.3.5 Detection limits

As noted above, the theoretical number of ASV can be very large, and many are not detectable due to the ASV complexities and limits of current technologies. First of all, multiple ASV may be present in any given tissue sample, i.e. a mixture of different ASV. Different ASV may involve different or the same sets of probes. Hence, the intensity values of individual probes reflect summations of all different ASV represented by the corresponding probes. Secondly, given the limited number of probes, the theoretical number of detectable ASV is also much smaller. Suppose that we have a perfectly designed probe for each exon. Hence, in the absence of any sample mixture, we can detect 2^{N-2} possible combinations of individual probes. Hence, many ASV would not be differentiable, based upon these perfect probes. Thirdly, typical probes and their hybridization measurements are subject to a host of technical variations. The magnitude of these variations, coupled with the natural sample variations, would impose limits on the detection of ASV. The full recognition of these limits, and many others, would require careful use of statistical methods to extract pertinent information relating to ASV, and, more importantly, cautious interpretation of any positive findings.

8.4 An example

For illustration purposes, here is an example of how a bioinformatic approach is used to predict ASV that differ between normal cerebellum and medulloblastomas (Fan et al., 2006). This dataset consists of GeneChip® Hu6800 expression array data from 69 medulloblastoma samples and four cerebellum samples as normal controls. Among the medulloblastomas samples, 42 are from non-metastatic tumours and 27 are from metastatic tumours. There are 7129 probe sets in the Hu6800 expression array. Each probe set includes 20 pairs of perfect and mismatched probes, each of which target different segments of a gene. As noted above, this array technology is designed for assessing abundance of transcripts, without optimizing ASV assessments. Nevertheless, one can utilize such data for an exploratory analysis of ASV.

From the design perspective, this study may be considered as the unmatched two-group comparison. Utilizing the general framework described in Section 8.3.3, we attempted to identify ASV that may partially explain the difference between medulloblastomas and normal cerebellum. First, we predicted splice variants between the normal cerebellum and medulloblastoma tumour samples, including both non-metastatic and metastatic tumours. Operationally, in this step, using a significance level of 0.05 in the t-tests, we identified 10,838 pseudo-exons out of a total of 142,580 (7129×20) probes representing the 7129 probe sets on the Hu6800 GeneChip®. A schematic illustration of the probe configuration is shown in Fig. 8.3. In the second step, we compared the difference in expression values between the two groups for each of the pseudo-exons. The histogram of Z-scores from this comparison is shown in Fig. 8.4. By the significance threshold of Z-score = 4.8 (equivalent to one false positive), we discovered 811 pseudo-exons, which are derived from 577 genes, to be significantly different between these two groups. Note that some genes had more than one selected pseudo-exon. A distribution of the number of pseudo-exons compared to the number of exons in a given gene is shown in Fig. 1.5, and the full list of genes can be found as a supplement to (Fan *et al.*, 2006).

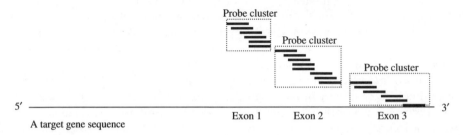

FIG. 8.3: An graphic illustration of probes within GeneChip®.

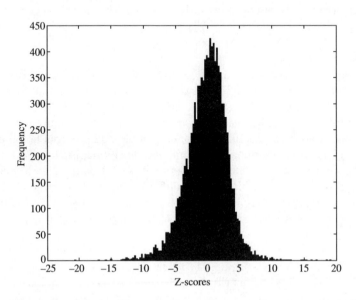

FIG. 8.4: Histogram of the Z-scores for comparison between cerebellum and medulloblastomas.

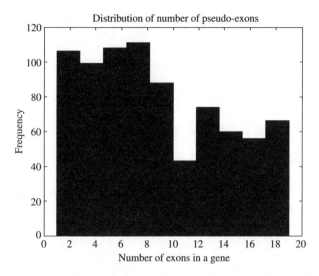

FIG. 8.5: Frequency of pseudo-exons by number of exons in a given gene.

Applying the PathwayAssist^{TM} software (http://www.ariadnegenomics.com/products/pathway.html), we searched the literature for pathways the 577 genes represent to shed light on the functions of these genes. The recognized pathways can be broadly grouped into either growth/differentiation or apoptosis-related pathways. For example, the MAPK, EGF, SAPK-JNK and PDGF pathways are involved in cellular growth and differentiation processes; and apoptosis, caspase, and TNF pathways relate to apoptosis.

When comparing metastatic to non-metastatic tumours, 13 genes were identified as having ASV that differed between the tumour types. Five of out of the 13 genes that we predict to have ASV were previously reported in the literature to have splice variants. They are nitric oxide synthase 1 (NOS1) (Wang et al., 1999), low density lipoprotein receptor (LDLR) (Kim et al., 1997), thrombopoietin (THPO) (Gurney et al., 1995), Down syndrome critical region gene 1 (DSCR1) (Fuentes et al., 1997), and paired box gene 2 (PAX2) (Tavassoli et al., 1997). This provides support that the methodology described can identify biologically significant ASV differences between tissue types.

8.5 Future directions

The general framework described above can be readily generalized to study various aspects of biological processes. For example, one aspect of a biological process is the dynamics of transcription related to that process over time. To investigate this property, one may design a time-course study, involving a serial collection of cellular samples at pre-set time points, $t_1, t_2, \ldots, t_n$. At every time point, one could use array technology to survey the transcriptome for various transcriptional signals. In this setting of a time-course study, one could adopt the same framework by replacing the disease status 'd_i' with the time variable or its transformation. The entire estimation and inference framework is readily applicable to dissect temporal changes in ASV. This design is particularly useful for studies involving cell lines. Its application to human studies is somewhat limited, largely due to sample availability over time.

Another use of this framework is to assess how a group of identified ASV candidates correlates with known ASV datasets. Statistically, one could apply this framework by bringing in the known ASV as a covariate, and then could assess how other transcript forms are associated with the covariate. This level of flexibility in modelling affords us the ability to focus on biological problem at hand. As we are postulating models, it is essential for data analysts to understand biological questions, processes, and experimental constraints, so that the model is appropriate for addressing scientific questions at hand. On the other hand, it is equally important for biologists to understand the quantitative framework, assumptions being made, and to utilize this knowledge for the appropriate interpretation of results. Together, bioinformatics specialists, working with biologists, can postulate sensible models and systematically analyse large data sets to evaluate different alternative splicing variants in cancer biology.

References

Barash, Y., Dehan, E., Krupsky, M., Franklin, W., Geraci, M., Friedman, N., and Kaminski, N. (2004). Comparative analysis of algorithms for signal quantitation from oligonucleotide microarrays. *Bioinformatics*, **20**, 839–846.

Brown, P. O. and Botstein, D. (1999). Exploring the new world of the genome with dna microarrays. *Nature Genetics*, **21**, 33–37.

Brown, P. O. and Hartwell, L. (1998). Genomics and human disease – variations on variation. *Nature Genetics*, **18**, 91–93.

Fan, W., Khalid, N., Hallahan, A. R., Olson, J. M., and Zhao, L. P. (2006). A statistical method for predicting splice variants between two groups of samples using genechip expression array data. *Theoretical Biology and Medical Modelling*, **3**, 19.

Fuentes, J. J., Pritchard, M. A., and Estivill, X. (1997). Genomic organization, alternative splicing, and expression patterns of the dscr1 (down syndrome candidate region 1) gene. *Genomics*, **44**, 358–361.

Gurney, A. L., Kuang, W. J., Xie, M. H., Malloy, B. E., Eaton, D. L., and de Sauvage, F. J. (1995). Genomic structure, chromosomal localization, and conserved alternative splice forms of thrombopoietin. *Blood*, **85**, 981–988.

Hodges, D. and Bernstein, S. I. (1994). Genetic and biochemical analysis of alternative rna splicing. *Advances in Genetics*, **31**, 207–281.

Kim, D. H., Magoori, K., Inoue, T. R., Mao, C. C., Kim, H. J., Suzuki, H., Fujita, T., Endo, Y., Saeki, S., and Yamamoto, T. T. (1997). Exon/intron organization, chromosome localization, alternative splicing, and transcription units of the human apolipoprotein e receptor 2 gene. *Journal of Biological Chemistry*, **272**, 8498–8504.

Liang, K.-Y. and Zeger, S. L. (1986). Longitudinal data analysis using generalized linear models. *Biometrika*, **73**, 13–22.

Matsubara, K. and Okubo, K. (1993). Identification of new genes by systematic analysis of cdnas and database construction. *Current Opinion in Biotechnology*, **4**, 672–677.

Mockler, T. C., Chan, S., Sundaresan, A., Chen, H., Jacobsen, S. E., and Ecker, J. R. (2005). Applications of dna tiling arrays for whole-genome analysis. *Genomics*, **85**, 1–15.

Sorensen, A. B., Warming, S., Fuchtbauer, E.-M., and Pedersen, F. S. (2002). Alternative splicing, expression, and gene structure of the septin-like putative proto-oncogene sint1. *Gene*, **285**, 79–89.

Tavassoli, K., Ruger, W., and Horst, J. (1997). Alternative splicing in pax2 generates a new reading frame and an extended conserved coding region at the carboxy terminus. *Human Genetics*, **279**, 371–375.

Venables, J. P. (2006). Unbalanced alternative splicing and its significance in cancer. *Bioessays*, **28**, 378–86.

Wang, Y., Newton, D. C., and Marsden, P. A. (1999). Neuronal nos: gene structure, mrna diversity, and functional relevance. *Critical Reviews in Neurobiology*, **13**, 21–43.

INDEX

Affymetrix, xi, 26, 28–30, 43, 57, 64, 67, 70, 180, 181, 184, 186,
Allelic imbalance (AI), 52
Alternative splice variants (ASV), 180, 182,
Amplification, 25, 28–30, 33–35, 44, 47, 70, 72, 78–80, 84, 85, 90–92, 97, 107, 108, 117, 124,
Anova, 124, 128, 149,
Armitage trend test, 9, 14,
Array-CGH, 26, 29, 43, 81, 82, 89, 90, 92, 94, 96, 97
ArrayExpress, 161,
Artifacts, copy number profiling, 43, 46
Association analysis, 168, 169, 185,
ASV, 180–190

Background intensity, 88, 116,
Bibliosphere, 134
BioPax, 136
Bisulphite conversion, 106, 107, 110, 111, 113, 114,
Bisulphite sequencing, 106, 107, 110, 112, 128
   cloned, 106, 107
   direct, 106, 107, 110, 112, 128
Bonferroni correction, 15

Cancer Outlier Profile Analysis (COPA), 160
CBS, 31, 33
cDNA array, 180
CERP/CART, 139
CGH microarray, 81, 92
CGH-Plotter, 84, 91, 94
CGHweb, 33
Chi-squared test, 8, 10
Circular Binary Segmentation (CBS), 31
Classification, 12, 60, 81, 104, 118–124, 128, 132, 139–142, 145, 151, 152,
Classification and Regression Tree (CART), 12, 139
Clinical endpoints, 55
CNV, 12, 37, 38, 44

Co-expression, 145, 160, 161, 163, 167–169
Colorectal cancer, 1, 2, 12, 14, 18, 19, 56, 105, 123, 125, 126
Common-disease common-variant hypothesis, 1, 2, 12
Comparative Genomic Hybridization (CGH), 26, 79
Copy number, 25–48, 52–61, 65–74, 78–98, 117
   Allele specific, 28, 57, 67, 68
Copy number aberration (CNA), 25, 33, 36, 37
Copy number variation (CNV), 36, 38, 43, 48, 58, 72, 81, 82, 93, 98
COSMIC, 54
CpG, 102, 103, 105–128
   CpG island, 103, 107
Cytogenic data, 177
Cytoscape, 133, 134

Data pre-processing, 105
dChipSNP, 57, 61, 66, 67
Deletion, 4, 25, 30, 34–38, 41–44, 47, 48, 54, 67, 71, 78–81, 84, 90–92, 97,
Differential display, 80
Differential expression, 46, 82, 91, 160–164, 167–169, 174
Differential methylation hybridization (DMH), 107
Digital Karyotyping, 28, 29
DMH, 107, 114–117
DNAcopy, R package, 31

EASE/DAVID, 137,
Entrez Gene, 161, 168
Epigenetics, 102
Estimating equation, 185, 186
Exhaustive search, 120, 122, 123
Exon, 177–189
   Exon array, 181, 183
   Exon skipping, 178

False Discovery Rate (FDR), 15, 134,
False Positives, 31, 124

Familial risk, 1
Fatigo, 137
FCS, 136, 137, 142, 147
FDR, 15, 134, 138, 149,
Feature selection, 119–122
Fisher criterion, 120–123, 128
Fisher's exact test, 6, 8, 9, 44, 137, 143, 144, 169
Functional class scoring (FCS), 136, 137

G-banding, 79, 80
GenBank, 161
Gene conversion, 52, 55
Gene fusions, 44
Gene Ontology, 4, 85, 93, 97, 135
Gene-environment interaction, 9, 11
Gene-gene interaction, 12, 147
Gene-level-paradigm, 138, 140, 141, 142, 147, 152
GeneChip, 11, 28, 180, 181, 187, 188
Generalized probe model, 177
Generalized singular value decomposition (GSVD), 94–96
GenMAPP, 133, 134
Genomatix, 133
Genome Topography Scan (GTS), 40, 43, 44
Genome-wide association study, 2
Genomic Identification of Significant Targets in Cancer (GISTIC), 40
Genotype, 3, 4–14, 53–68,
  Informative, 60
  Non-informative, 60
GEO, 161
GO, 97, 98, 135, 168
GoMiner, 137
GSEA, 136, 137, 142, 146, 147
GSVD, 94, 95

Haplotype, 3, 4, 10, 11
Hardy-Weinberg equilibrium, 6
Hidden Markov Model (HMM), 33, 53, 61
Hidden states, 61, 63, 65, 70, 90
Hierarchical Clustering, 47, 163
HMM, 53, 61, 65–68, 70
Hybridization, 26, 28, 31, 36, 79, 82, 84, 88, 107, 108, 116, 185
Hybridization intensities, 108, 115–117
Hypermethylated, 103, 108, 128
Hypomethylated, 103, 108

iCNA, R package, 44
Illumina, 28, 57
Incomplete conversion, 110, 113
Informative genotype, 60
Ingenuity Pathway Analysis, 133
Intensity value, 67, 82, 161, 180, 184–186,
Interaction, 9, 11, 97, 103, 135, 142, 161, 163, 170
  Gene-environment, 9, 11
  Gene-gene, 12, 134, 147
Interpolation, 96, 97
Intragenic CNA, 29, 44
Intron, 44, 178, 181

Kaplan-Meier analysis, 127
Knudson's Two-hit Hypothesis, 53, 54, 103

Likelihood, 10, 31, 39, 63, 122, 171, 185
Linear model, 116, 185
Linkage disequilibrium, 2, 3
Logistic regression, 10–12, 123, 125
Loss of Heterozygosity (LOH), 52, 60, 65
Loss of imprinting, 105
LPE, 134, 143

MAQC Consortium, 139
Marker panel, 123, 125, 126
Markov property, 62
Matinspector, 134
Messenger RNA (mRNA), 78, 80, 177
Meta-analysis, 139, 164, 167, 169–171, 174
MetaCore, 85, 133, 135
Metamap, 164
Methylation, 9, 29, 103, 105, 107, 109, 110, 115
  odds, 44, 109, 118, 119
  rate, 107–110, 113, 114–118, 126, 128
Methylation analysis, 104, 107, 110, 128
  global, 106, 107, 113, 135
Methylation sensitive restriction, 106, 107
Methylation-specific PCR, 108
MintViewer, 134
Mixed Model Analysis, 134
MM probe (mismatch probe), 57
MMA Method, 138
Moderated t-test, 134
Multiple Myeloma, 55
Multiple Sample Analysis (MSA), 40
Mutation, 1, 6, 11, 15, 18, 37, 39, 52, 54, 104, 140, 145

Index

Natural selection, 55
Nearest Neighbour (NN), 61
Non-informative genotype, 53, 60
Non-negative matrix factorization (NMF), 47
Non-specific binding, 27, 57
Normalisation (SNP arrays), 28, 53, 57
Normalization, 57, 68, 88, 89, 109–116, 186, 187

Odds Ratio, 44, 109, 126, 169
Oligonucleotide probes, designing, 81, 181
Oncomine, 160–163, 167–170
Oncomine Cluster Signatures, 167–169
Oncomine Concepts Map, 163, 167–170
ORA, 136, 142
Osprey, 133, 134
Over-expression, 83–85, 92
Over-representation analysis (ORA), 133, 136

p-value, 9, 12, 14, 15, 39, 125, 126, 137, 143, 144, 164
PAM, 139
Pathway, 5, 85, 98, 132, 140–142, 145
   analysis, 12, 132–140, 142, 145
   classification, 142
   level paradigm, 152
   signatures, 152
Pathway Pattern Extraction, 143–146
Pathway Studio, 133
PCA, 46, 47, 121
Permutation test, 92, 93
PM probe (perfect match probe), 57, 58
Polygenic model, 1, 2, 11
Polysomy, 55
Population stratification, 6, 13, 14, 17
Pre-processing, 105
Principle Component Analysis (PCA), 46, 47, 120, 121
Probabilistic model, 61
Probe intensity, 115, 116, 186

Q-value, 4, 162–164
Quantile-quantile plot, 7

r^2, 3, 7–9,
Random Forest, 139, 146,
RB1, 53, 54
Receiver operating characteristic (ROC), 31, 32, 124,

Receiver operating characteristic (ROC), application to copy number aberration, 44, 90, 124
Recombination, 13, 17, 18, 38, 44, 52, 55
   Homologous, 55
RefSeq, 161
Regions with Same Boundary (RSB), 60
Regression model, 10, 11, 125, 126, 128
Remote sample, 104, 109
Representational Oligonucleotide Microarray Analysis (ROMA), 28
Restriction Fragment Length Polymorphism (RFLP), 53
Retinoblastoma, 53, 54
RFLP, 53, 56
ROC, 31, 32, 90, 124
ROMA, 28

SAGE, 28, 29, 80
SAM, 148, 149
Sample impurity, 65
SBML, 136
Segmentation, 31-35, 38, 46, 90, 94
Self-Organizing Maps (SOM), 134
Serial analysis of gene expression (SAGE), 80
Significance Analysis of Microarray (SAM), 134
Significance Testing for Aberrant Copy-Number (STAC), 39
Single nucleotide polymorphism (SNP), xi, 2, 3, 53, 104
Singular value decomposition (SVD), 94, 136, 137
SLEPR, 143, 144, 146–149
SNP, 11, 3–15, 20, 28–30, 34, 36, 39, 43, 44, 52, 53, 56–74, 149
SNP array (SNP genotyping array), 28, 52, 53, 57, 61, 149
SOM, 134
Spectral karyotyping, 80
Splicing, 177–179
STAC, 39, 40
Stanford Microarray Database, 161
Statistical significance, 14, 91, 137, 162
Steerable gene shaving, 95, 96
STKE, 132
Student's t-test, 122
Support Vector Machine (SVM), 119–123
Survival analysis, 127
SVD, 94, 136, 137
SVM, 119–123, 125, 128
SVMs, 120, 122

T-Profiler, 137
Tagging, 5, 11
TDT, 13
The HapMap project (The International HapMap project), 3, 13, 18, 56
Tissue classification, 118
TP53, 14, 55, 72
Transcript abundance, 187
Translocations, 25, 44, 48
Transmission disequilibrium test (TDT), 13
TSG, 53, 54, 72
Tumour suppressor gene (TSG), 54, 72
Two group design, 182

Under-expression, 84–86, 164, 171
UniGene, 161
Uniparental disomy, 55, 67, 71, 72, 74

VisANT, 135

WGSA, 28
Whole Genome Sampling Assay (WGSA), 28
WPS, 133, 134, 137, 143, 144, 146,